CHEMISTRY JOB ASSISTANT

AN ULTIMATE SOLUTION FOR YOUR CAREER

JULIA JOHNSON

1. Introduction

Acquiring a degree in chemistry opens a multitude of doors for graduates for a variety of educational or professional opportunities. From chemical engineer to lecturer to pharmacologist to chemist, career opportunities are vast, to say the least. A chemistry degree is a golden key that grants access to seemingly infinite professional possibilities.

If you know you want to pursue a career in chemistry, but you're not positive on what your finish line looks like, **Chemistry Job Assistant** is a perfect book that will show you a way to equip yourself with a competitor for professional roles.

Chemistry graduates are in demand from companies carrying out scientific research. Depending on which topics they specialized in during their course, students might find a career working for pharmaceutical or metallurgical companies, or providing analysis for commercial laboratories. The criminal justice system needs chemistry graduates to work as forensic scientists, providing evidence for the courts using state-of-the-art techniques. Outside of the lab there are many opportunities for chemists.

Graduates can become consultants in fields like the environment and sustainability, offering insights into how organizations should adhere to environmental regulations. A chemistry degree also gives graduates the scientific insight to become a patent attorney, with further study into intellectual property law. Many chemistry graduates opt for a career in teaching at school or university level, and others continue to study for an MSc or PhD.

In this book every sectors and different terms, instrumentations of chemistry and their impacts are discussed. Here also different job sectors of chemistry and as chemist your responsibilities in there are also discussed. So this book will you help to boost up your confidence and assist you to build up a sustainable career in chemistry

1.1. Definition of Chemistry

Chemistry is a sub discipline of science that deals with the study of matter and the substances that constitute it. It also deals with the properties of these substances and the reactions undergone by them to form new substances. Chemistry primarily focuses on atoms, ions, and molecules which, in turn, make up elements and compounds. These chemical species tend to interact with each other through chemical bonds. It is important to note that the interactions between matter and energy are also studied in the field of chemistry.

All of the objects around you this book, your pen or pencil, and the things of nature such as rocks, water, plant and animal substances constitute the matter of the universe. Each of the particular kinds of matter, such as a certain kind of paper or plastic or metal, is referred to as a material. We can define chemistry as the science of the composition and structure of materials and of the changes that materials undergo.

One chemist may hope that by understanding certain materials, he or she will be able to find a cure for a disease or a solution for an environmental ill. Another chemist may simply want to understand a phenomenon. Because chemistry deals with all materials, it is a subject of enormous breadth. It would be difficult to exaggerate the influence of chemistry on modern science and technology or on our ideas about our planet and the universe.

1.2. Relationship between Chemistry and Other Branches of Science

'Science' can be defined as the systematic study of the natural universe, its structure, and everything it encompasses. Due to the immensity of the natural universe, science has been divided into several disciplines that deal with certain aspects of the universe. The three primary subcategories of science under which these disciplines can be grouped are:

The Formal Sciences: Involves the study of the language disciplines that concern formal systems. Examples of scientific disciplines that fall under this category include logic and mathematics. Can be thought of as the "language of science".

The Natural Sciences: Involves the study of natural phenomena through experiments and observations. Chemistry, physics, and biology fall under this category of science.

The Social Sciences: Involves the study of human societies and the relationships between the humans that dwell in these societies. Examples of scientific disciplines that fall under this category include psychology, sociology, and economics.

2.   Chemistry as a Career

As if choosing the degree weren't hard enough, you're eventually going to have to choose a career path which holds its own circus of questions. A chemistry degree is a golden key that grants access to seemingly infinite professional possibilities.

Take time and think about your experiences. What did you enjoy most about your studies? What experiments or research truly intrigued you? What bridges the divide between who you are as a person and who you are a student? If you had the chance to do an internship, what did you value about it? Who did you meet?

Start developing a sense of what you want. Look at your network. See who among your contacts might have access to companies, laboratories or roles that fit your "passion point." Use your honed study skills to become an expert of the search. The key is to analyze the market and find a way to turn yourself into a category expert that will easily differentiate yourself from all other candidates seeking a position in your chosen category."

Become a student of your quest to find fit, and invite input starting with your own sense of what you want and then expanding out to your network.

After completing the necessary educational requirements, a professional in chemistry can go for the following careers in the field of chemistry:

Research & Development

- Research and Product Development
- Cheminformatics
- Engineering and Technology
- Crystallography
- Pigments, Inks, and Dyes
- Laboratory, Project and Industrial Management
- Management
- Project Management

Quality Control/Regulatory

- Toxicology
- Safety and Health
- Toxic or Hazardous Waste Management
- Quality Assurance
- Quality control

Support

- Information Management Specialist
- Human Resources
- Public Information
- Support and Communication
- Technical Communication

Sales/Marketing

- Technical Sales and Marketing

Manufacturing

- Process and Formulation Chemistry

Law and Policy

- Law
- Public Information
- Regulation of Affairs
- Policy
- Social Impact

Military & Law Enforcement

- Military Science & Technology
- Forensic Science

Higher Education

- Professional Staff
- Basic Research
- Cheminformatics
- Professor
- Information Management

2.1. Careers in Chemistry

If you have a particular interest in or aptitude for chemistry, or if you hold or are currently working towards a chemistry degree, you may wish to find out about potential careers in the industry. Chemistry jobs vary in nature, salary, and required qualifications; the information and list below is intended to help you to judge the right chemistry career for you.

- Analytical Chemist
- Chemical Engineer
- Chemistry Teacher
- Forensic Scientist
- Geochemist
- Hazardous Waste Chemist
- Materials Scientist
- Pharmacologist
- Toxicologist
- Water Chemist
- Ceramic Chemists
- Food Scientist
- Environmental Chemist
- Petroleum Chemist
- Medicinal Chemist

Analytical Chemist

Analytical chemists use their skills and expertise to analyze substances, identify what components are present and in what quantities, as well how these components may behave and react with one another. This can include the analysis of drugs, food and other products to determine effectiveness, quality and to ensure they are safe for human consumption or use.

Chemical Engineer

Chemical engineers are involved the design and development of new products from raw materials. They use their knowledge of chemical properties and reactions to transform materials from one state to another, for example making plastic from oil. Chemical engineers may work in almost any industry, assisting in the production of innovative, high-end products such as ultra-strong fabrics or biocompatible implants.

Chemistry Teacher

Chemistry teachers work in schools, colleges and universities passing on their knowledge of chemistry to the next generation, following a set curriculum and helping their students to pass and excel in their examinations. As well as a degree or equivalent qualification in chemistry, you may also require a teaching qualification in order to become a chemistry teacher.

Forensic Scientist

Forensic scientists search for and analyze forensic materials found at crime scenes, for example blood and other bodily fluids, hair, or non-biological substances such as paint. They are then able to present this evidence for use in legal investigations and courts of law. Forensic scientists may sometimes be called in to speak in court as experts in their field, to explain the evidence to the jury.

Geochemist

Geochemists study the physical and chemical properties of the Earth, particularly rocks and minerals. They use their knowledge to determine the make-up and distribution of rock and mineral components, and how these may affect the soil and water systems in which they are found. Geochemists may help to identify oil drill sites, improve water quality or determine how best to remove hazardous waste.

Hazardous Waste Chemist

Hazardous waste chemists deal with the management and safe relocation of hazardous materials (hence the common abbreviation 'hazmat'). They use their expertise to identify harmful chemical components in the air, water or soil, evaluate the danger they present and coordinate their removal and containment.

Materials Scientist

Materials scientists study man-made and natural substances to determine their properties, composition and how they could be transformed or combined to increase effectiveness or create new materials. By analyzing and experimenting with existing materials, materials scientists are able to enhance the way they are used and create new materials to better serve humanity's needs.

Pharmacologist

Pharmacologists undertake the development and testing of drugs, analyzing how they interact with biological systems. This is essential for ensuring that drugs are effective and safe for human use, and may involve the testing of drugs on animals or on human volunteers. Pharmacology roles are often lab-based and may involve non-standard hours in order to monitor ongoing experiments.

Toxicologist

Toxicologists, like pharmacologists, may study the effects of drugs on biological systems but also look at the effects of other substances, both natural and man-made. They work with and develop methodologies for determining harmful effects of substances, as well as how to judge correct dosages and therefore avoid them. As with pharmacology, toxicology roles are often lab-based and involve the monitoring of experiments and interpretation of results.

Water Chemist

Water chemists, as the name suggests, are concerned with analyzing and maintaining the quality and condition of water, essential for human life on Earth. This is a highly interdisciplinary field, so as well as chemistry you may also need knowledge of linked fields such as microbiology and geology. You may find similar roles under a variety of names, for example hydrologist or hydrogeologist.

Ceramic Chemists

Ceramic materials are materials having advanced properties such as high strength and thermal resistance. Ceramic Chemists put all their knowledge into developing such advanced ceramic materials which find usage in important industrial sectors such as Aerospace industry, cutting tool manufacturing industry and insulation industry. Further, it is because of the wide range of applications which ceramics find in different industrial sectors, such as the ones mentioned above, that ceramic chemists always remain high in demand. Also, ceramic chemists enjoy a good pay scale and thus, lead a professional life of fulfillment.

Food Scientist

Food items are mostly composed of organic compounds thus organic chemists have a good scope of employment as food scientists in the food industry. Further, food scientists are required to use their vast knowledge to enhance the nutritional value of the different food items which are used for consumption. Not only this, they also analyze the food items and ensure that they are safe and healthy for people to consume. Further, food scientists get employed at a handsome pay scale in all types of food processing industries both in the private as well as government sector. It is only because of eminent food scientists that we can consume packaged and canned food items with the trust of safety.

Environmental Chemist

The alarming rise in the levels of environmental pollution is a cause of concern for the entire world. The soil, the air, the water and all other constituents of the environment are being polluted by chemicals and other toxic substances which are being released into them. As a result of the increased pollution levels, the entire world is dealing with numerous environmental problems such as global warming, ozone layer depletion and rise in the sea level. To throw light on the risks associated with these problems, environmental chemists deal with the study of the impact of the pollutants on the environment and biodiversity. They also develop various techniques and technologies to bring a reduction in environmental pollution such as waste management techniques and developing alternatives for non-biodegradable materials like plastic. Moreover, as environmental pollution and problems form major concerning issues which need to be addressed at priority by the entire humanity, environmental chemists always remain high in demand and thus, have a promising career ahead of them.

Petroleum Chemist

Petroleum and its products find important application in the industrial and household sector such as heat, electricity and energy generation in automobile engines. Petroleum Chemists deal with everything which is associated with petroleum and its products. If you are involved at working in this branch, then you are required to devise innovative ways to make more efficient and judicious use of petroleum, exploring new petroleum reserves and developing new petroleum products are some examples of tasks which you would need to perform. Furthermore, the professional journey of petroleum chemists begins by undertaking rigorous training in the respective companies, under the guidance of experts. Once petroleum chemists complete their training and gain the required amount of experience in their field, they soar high in professional success with an attractive pay scale.

Medicinal Chemist

As discussed above, most of the medicines used in the healthcare industry are derived from organic compounds. Thus, organic chemists get employed in the medical industry, as medicinal chemists. It is by applying their immense knowledge about organic compounds that they synthesize novel medicines and drugs for the treatment of various diseases and ailments. Along with this, they also conduct wide scale research on improving the derivation techniques and processes of various medicines. Moreover, the healthcare industry is one of the most basic and essentially required industries for the survival of mankind. Thus, medicinal chemists are always high in demand and also enjoy a good level of job security.

Entry-Level Jobs of Chemistry

Kick-off your chemistry career in one of these exciting entry-level positions:

- Lab Tech
- Research Chemist
- Assistant Chemist
- Process Chemist
- Entry-Level Pharmaceutical Chemist

Internships of Chemistry

Gain insight, experience and industry connections by applying for a chemistry internship. Here are a few popular internships with roles around the country:

- Chemical Information Intern
- Pharmaceutical Intern
- Undergraduate Researcher
- Laboratory Technician

Most of the chemistry jobs listed above will require you to have some level of qualification in chemistry, whether that's a bachelor's degree, master's degree or PhD. Some roles you may be able to pursue with a qualification in a related field, for example biology, environmental science or pharmacology.

Many chemistry jobs are lab-based, though not all - a number of roles may include field work, office work, or even teaching in a school, university or other academic environment. More senior roles can involve people management, liaison with businesses and management of departments and budgets.

Further study

Many chemistry graduates undertake further study at Masters or PhD level to increase their knowledge of one of the branches studied during their degree, such as organic, inorganic, physical or analytical chemistry.

You may also specialize in areas of applied chemistry, such as cheminformatics or biochemistry, or develop knowledge in an area where chemistry graduates may be in demand, for example, forensic nanotechnology and forensic investigation.

Further study is highly valued by employers, particularly within scientific and technical fields, as you'll develop more advanced theoretical knowledge and practical sector-specific skills.

2.2. Importance of Chemistry as a Career

Chemistry is an incredibly fascinating field of study. Because it is so fundamental to our world, chemistry plays a role in everyone's lives and touches almost every aspect of our existence in some way. Chemistry is essential for meeting our basic needs of food, clothing, shelter, health, energy, and clean air, water, and soil. Chemical technologies enrich our quality of life in numerous ways by providing new solutions to problems in health, materials, and energy usage. Thus, studying chemistry is useful in preparing us for the real world.

Chemistry is often referred to as the central science because it joins together physics and mathematics, biology and medicine, and the earth and environmental sciences. Knowledge of the nature of chemicals and chemical processes therefore provides insights into a variety of physical and biological phenomena. Knowing something about chemistry is worthwhile because it provides an excellent basis for understanding the physical universe, we live in. For better or for worse, everything is chemical!

The behavior of atoms, molecules, and ions determines the sort of world we live in, our shapes and sizes, and even how we feel on a given day. Chemists who understand these phenomena are very well equipped to tackle problems faced by our modern society. On any given day, a chemist may be studying the mechanism of the recombination of DNA molecules, measuring the amount of insecticide in drinking water, comparing the protein content of meats, developing a new antibiotic, or analyzing a moon rock. To design a synthetic fiber, a life-saving drug, or a space capsule requires a knowledge of chemistry. To understand why an autumn leaf turns red, or why a diamond is hard, or why soap gets us clean, requires, first, a basic understanding of chemistry.

It may be obvious to you that a chemistry background is important if you plan to teach chemistry or to work in the chemical industry developing chemical commodities such as polymeric materials, pharmaceuticals, flavorings, preservatives, dyestuffs, or fragrances. You may also be aware that chemists are frequently employed as environmental scientists, chemical oceanographers, chemical information specialists, chemical engineers, and chemical salespersons. However, it may be less obvious to you that a significant knowledge of chemistry is often required in a number of related professions including medicine, pharmacy, medical technology, nuclear medicine, molecular biology, biotechnology, pharmacology, toxicology, paper science, pharmaceutical science, hazardous waste management, art conservation, forensic science and patent law. Thus, a chemistry degree can be effectively combined with advanced work in other fields which may lead, for example, to work in higher management (sometimes with an M.B.A.), the medical field (with a medical degree), or in the patent field (possibly with a law degree).

Studying chemistry also puts one in an excellent position to choose from a wide variety of useful, interesting and rewarding careers. A person with a bachelor's level education in chemistry is well prepared to assume professional positions in industry, education, or public service. A chemistry degree also serves as an excellent foundation for advanced study in a number of related areas. The list of career possibilities for people with training in chemistry is long and varied. Even in times when unemployment rates are high, the chemist remains one of the most highly sought after and employed scientists

It is often observed that today's graduate, unlike the graduate of a generation ago, should anticipate not a single position with one employer or in one industry, but rather many careers. You will be well prepared for this future if, in your college years, you take advantage of the opportunity to become broadly educated, to learn to be flexible and to be a creative problem solver. Knowledge and skills gained in your college courses may be directly applicable in your first job, but science and technology change at a rapid pace. You will keep up and stay ahead if you graduate with the skills and self-discipline to pursue a lifetime of learning. Since chemistry provides many of these skills and is a fundamental driver in the business and commerce sector of our society, chemists are likely to remain in continual demand.

3. Job Sectors of Chemistry

A chemistry graduate has a huge job opportunity in different sectors. Chemists typically work in plants that manufacture products formed from chemical reactions, such as pharmaceuticals, oil, cosmetics and fertilizers etc. They conduct laboratory research to find effective ways to optimize production processes, improve production safety and product quality, and reduce environmental pollution. Chemists can also find job opportunities at research and development facilities.

Some of the job sectors are listed below

1. Pharmaceutical industry
2. Paint industry
3. Textile industry
4. Food and beverage industry
5. Standard or in-house Laboratory
6. Paper industry
7. Cement industry
8. Personal Care industry
9. Fertilizers industry
10. Educational Institution
11. Petrochemical industry

3.1. Pharmaceutical Industry

Pharmaceutical industry, the discovery, development, and manufacture of drugs and medications (pharmaceuticals) by public and private organizations. It discovers, develops, produces, and markets drugs or pharmaceutical drugs for use as medications to be administered (or self-administered) to patients, with the aim to cure them, vaccinate them, or alleviate the symptoms.

The Pharmaceutical Chemist performs set up, calibration, operation, and maintenance of laboratory test equipment. Performs assigned work in a timely and safe manner conforming to regulatory, company, and compendial requirements. The Pharmaceutical Chemist performs routine and non-routine quality control testing of raw materials, in process, residual, finished product, and stability testing within the framework of the site policies and cGMP regulations.

A chemistry graduate can work at Quality control department and Research & Development department in pharmaceutical industry. They provide higher attractive salary to chemist.

3.2. Paint Industry

Paint Industry is also a goldmine for Chemistry graduate. They offer an attractive salary to chemist. Here chemist works as a quality tester and as a researcher of new product. The Chemist for the Innovation Lab develops or improves formulations in the area of consumer and industrial products (e.g. coatings, adhesives, sealants, paints, inks, cosmetics, cleaners, food and beverages etc.) Performs analytical testing using a variety of technologies possibly including HPLC, GPC, GC/MS, SEM-EDX, FTIR, NMR and UV-Vis spectroscopy. Has learned multiple methodologies and techniques to be able to maximally contribute to the organization. Executes projects of moderate complexity in support of client needs. Types of projects include: Product formulation and development, product deformulation, polymer characterization, failure analysis and problem solving, stability and performance testing.

3.3. Textile Industry

You may think of the textile industry involving a series of spinning, weaving, dyeing, and finishing a range of products from bathroom towels to winter sweaters. Indeed, the textile industry process is a complex one involving many steps from taking raw fibers and turning them into a product that consumers can use and enjoy.

The use of chemistry can add special properties to fabrics that live up to the claims brands project like keeping you cool in the heat or absorbing sweat. Textile chemists have an understanding of the textile manufacturing process, such as the different types of fibers used, as well as the knowledge to apply chemistry principles to that process. Textile chemists generally work in three areas: Dyeing and finishing chemistry, Fiber and polymer chemistry, Blending different textile materials

Textile chemistry can be found throughout the textile industry in research and development, environmental testing, and dyeing and finishing in a wide range of chemistry types ranging from surface chemistry to organic chemistry

3.4. Food and Beverage Industry

A food chemist is an individual whose job is to perform research in order to develop and improve food and beverages. They have to perform tests using a number of methods that includes merging natural as well as synthetic food materials. They also have to analyze the sensory effects of food. It is the job of a food chemist to develop and implement policies and practicing procedures in regards to the decorum of the laboratory. They have to create all the required correspondence and highlight the progress of various projects. He may also have to lead a team in order to administer tests and analyze food to achieve the goals set by clients.

3.5. Standard or In-house Laboratory

In standard or in-house laboratory like Intertek, SGS Ltd. chemist work as a researcher. They have to conduct all allotted tests as per methods and SOP. Responsible for sample breakdown, extraction, preparation and instrumentation. Prepare initial test report and verify accuracy of test results. Ensure all assigned tests are completed within stipulated timeline. Keep all necessary records of the tests conducted. Maintain stock records and monitor the consumables. Maintain all QC parameters as per SOP/guideline and update daily QC. Maintain equipment performance and up-to-date calibration records.

3.6. Paper Industry

Pulp and paper chemists focus their work on the industrial paper-making process. Much of their job is geared towards improving efficiency, making the process more cost-effective and environmentally friendly.

A chemist starting in the field will likely spend most of his or her time in the lab. However, unless that chemist's work remains in research, more and more time will be spent in mill and plant facilities. Because their work is always geared toward the end product, experienced paper chemists, including those whose jobs are in the marketing department, say they spend a lot of time knee deep in paper fiber and sludge, trying to determine how to improve paper and the paper-making process. The paper industry employs chemists at pulp and paper companies, paper chemicals suppliers, and rosin chemicals makers. Consumer products manufacturers and specialty suppliers such as felt manufacturers also hire chemists. Engineering firms and environmental management companies employ chemists to work on their contracts with the paper industry.

3.7. Cement Industry

In cement industry chemists normally maintain quality parameters that meet the necessary requirements outlined by ASTM, AASHTO, State DOT s and customer requests. Provide quality and process interpretation for the clinker through microscopy in polished samples. Calibrate, maintain and certify instrumentation and analytical equipment. Maintain analytical equipment calibration and certification. Provide training for new employees or new techniques for existing employees. Ensures a safe work environment and safe working procedures are developed and maintained.

Chemists are highly paid in this sector. They work in production and quality control department.

3.8. Personal Care Industry

The personal care industry develops and manufactures products such as cosmetics, soaps, detergents, and more toiletries products, which are used for personal hygiene and beautification.

Personal care chemists work to understand the chemical and physical processes that describe how the raw ingredients work, how they affect each other, and how they affect the manufacturing process. They may design and manufacture new ingredients or combine and modify existing ingredients in new ways to create new products. Therefore, they need to make sure that desirable properties are maintained when ingredients are changed (due to changes in price or availability), and they are continually trying to develop better and more cost-effective products.

3.9. Fertilizer Industry

In fertilizer industry a chemistry student works as a scientist or quality control chemist and a production chemist.

Chemists help to establish the most cost-effective methods to produce product. Chemists may conduct tests to determine the chemical composition of the raw materials. They use this information to determine the proportions in which the raw materials can be mixed to increase fertilizer yields while maintaining product quality. If a chemical reaction along the production line takes a long time to occur, the chemist uses expertise to devise a solution, such as inducing a suitable chemical catalyst. They also maintain environmentally sustainable production activities.

3.10. Educational Institution

Working as a teacher at any school, college or university is fascinating. A Chemistry teacher is an educator who works in a school, college or university and teaches student basic, intermediate and advanced chemistry, all the while ensuring that their students are well-grounded in general scientific concepts and methods. They also demonstrate techniques and supervise students in laboratory experiments. The main role of a chemistry teacher is to teach different aspects of the subject at the level he is teaching, let students do various chemical experiments so that they get practical knowledge as it is a very important part of chemistry, let the students know of all the safety procedures to be followed, give them assignments, grade them and let them do various projects.

3.11. Petrochemical Industry

Petrochemicals are chemicals derived from petroleum or natural gas. They are an essential part of the chemical industry as the demand for synthetic materials grows continually and plays a major part in today's economy and society. Petrochemicals are used to manufacture thousands of different products that people use daily, including plastics, medicines, cosmetics, furniture, appliances, electronics, solar power panels, and wind turbines.

It's important to note that the biggest concern about fossil fuel use is from combustion, turning these hydrocarbons into carbon dioxide and water. So while there are environmental concerns about petrochemical manufacturing of plastics, it doesn't lead to a significant release of greenhouse gases that can cause climate change. For example, the plastic manufacturing is capturing the carbon in an inert form (the plastic) and not releasing it to the atmosphere.

Petrochemicals are derived from hydrocarbons such as propane, ethane, butane, or other components separated from crude oil and natural gas liquids. Naphtha - a mixture of flammable liquid hydrocarbons - is also important in the production of products made from petrochemicals. After being separated in some sort of distillation process, separated hydrocarbons can be fed to a manufacturing facility known as a cracker. This cracker works to break chemical bonds in hydrocarbon materials which allows them to be converted into more useful chemicals for production. One major petrochemical is ethylene, used to create polyethylene - one of the most important plastics in manufacturing.

4. Responsibilities

Chemists conduct experiments in labs in order to analyze substances, develop new products or improve existing ones. They may specialize in one or more areas, such as organic chemistry, inorganic chemistry, analytical chemistry, physical chemistry and biochemistry.

4.1. Responsibilities of a Chemist

- Prepare solutions by weighing ingredients and dissolving and diluting substances
- Analyze organic and inorganic compounds to determine their composition
- Conduct qualitative and quantitative experiments taking into account the volume and structure of ingredients
- Customize formulas and use different reagents to test chemical reactions
- Write technical reports of the test results
- Develop nonstandard tests for chemical products
- Maintain lab equipment and troubleshoot or report on malfunctions
- Refine chemical products to improve their quality
- Ensure compliance with laboratory health and safety guidelines
- Sterilize equipment and store materials in secure places

4.2. Responsibilities of a Chemistry Teacher

- Understanding the curriculum and developing schedules, lesson plans, and teaching methods that will help students cover the required content.
- Preparing and delivering lessons that are stimulating and clear.

- Educating students on lab safety and ensuring all experiments are carried out responsibly.
- Setting up tests, assignments, experiments, and grading students fairly.
- Ensuring appropriate resources and consultation times are available to students.
- Mentoring and providing support to student teachers.
- Attending staff and parent meetings, conferences, workshops, and other continuing education programs.
- Informing and preparing students for science fairs and expos.
- Handling various administration functions, which include updating student records and keeping track of lab supplies, tools, and equipment.
- Ensuring a safe, healthy classroom environment where learning can take place.

4.3. Responsibilities of QC Department

- Sampling adequately for testing purpose (physical, chemical and biological).
- Issuing release, reject or quarantine advice for each batch of raw and packaging materials.
- Assessment of the intermediate product for further processing.
- Assessment of the bulk products for their release, reprocess and reject etc.
- Storing keeping samples for each batch produced.
- Ensure precision and accuracy of all testing methods.
- Performing environmental monitoring cheeks calibration and standardization of laboratory equipment.
- Calibration and standardization of laboratory equipment.
- Control of laboratory reagents.
- Testing of any return goods.
- Analysis of complaint samples with their corresponding receiving samples.
- Monitoring batch wise full quality control test records with signature of the persons who performs the test.

4.4. Responsibilities of R&D Department

- Development of new products is usually the primary function of R&D
- Product maintenance is probably the most important secondary function of R&D
- Product enhancement helps keeping the company products ahead of the competition and extends the life of products
- The Quality R&D Interface as quality is a major issue and R&D are heavily involved in ensuring new products attain the required levels of quality
- Formulation development of new product.
- Formulation development of existing product.
- Ensuring product stability studies.
- In-vitro evaluation.
- Bio-equivalence studies.
- Process and equipment validation.
- Solving on-line production problems
- Analytical development.

4.5. Responsibilities of QA Department

- Ensuring fulfillment of regulatory requirements.
- Establishing specifications and control procedures for all starting materials, intermediates and finished products.
- Arranging quality audit visits to suppliers and self-inspection.
- Monitoring of the systems to ensure implementation of GMP & GLP in routine operation.
- Ensuring a suitable product quality review system exists.
- Establishing manufacturing methods and SOPs covering entire operations and their regular updating.

- In-Process checking of manufacturing operation of production area to ensure compliance with SOP.
- Ensure appropriate sampling of Bulk and Finished products as per sampling plan for QC analysis.
- Verify the rules of GMP & GLP, products safety and hygiene and also personal hygiene during work in progress.
- Train up the personnel as per cGMP and others guidelines.
- Perform and monitor the validation and calibration activities.
- Provide change over clearance in all areas of activities.
- Monitor temperature and humidity in all areas of the plant.
- Handle the non0conformities, customer complaints, change control and deviation management.
- Perform the management of retention samples.
- Review documents (SOPs, BMR, BPR, QC test report, tags, etc) of batches from time to time.

4.6. Responsibilities of Production Department

- Allocation of resources (Men/Machine/Materials) properly so as to ensure smooth production flow and delivery.
- Ensuring a smooth production flow / dynamically monitoring the production process and make necessary changes to achieve production based on the requirements.
- Achieving the production targets set by the management / orders given by the customers through optimum usage of the resources (men/materials/machine).
- Measuring and analyzing the current quality levels and taking necessary steps to improve and achieve the quality levels set by the management.
- Meeting the Quality requirements set by the customer and taking steps to exceed the quality requirements.
- Taking necessary steps to reduce costs – reducing defects / improving processes.

- Overall responsibility of delivering finished goods as per the customer's requirements.
- Ensuring 100% on-time delivery.
- Analysis of delays in deliveries and improvement from the current situations.
- Ensuring Safety of personnel and improving Morale of the employees - by implementing rewards and recognition for Attendance, Suggestion Schemes, Performance, etc.

5. Branches of Chemistry

There are 5 main branches of chemistry, every of that has several areas of study.

1. **Analytical Chemistry**
2. **Physical Chemistry**
3. **Organic Chemistry**
4. **Inorganic Chemistry**
5. **Biochemistry**

5.1. Analytical Chemistry

It is a branch of Chemistry that focusses on qualitative and quantitative methods to analyze properties of matter. In short, it deals with the analysis of chemicals. It has huge applications in chemical industries to maintain the quality of the final finished product. In real life, the steps in the analysis are separation, identification and finally quantification. In separation, we separate the constituents from the mixture. After isolating the desired sample, we identify its constituent by qualitative analysis. And finally, we estimate the concentration of analytes by quantitative analysis.

There are two classical methods used in Analytical Chemistry: qualitative and quantitative. The qualitative method involves identification of chemical constituents (atoms, molecules, ions etc.) in the substances. In the quantitative method determines the concentration of a substance in a given sample. With progress in science and technology, we are able to develop various instruments which can give better accuracy and precision.

Analytical Chemistry is not only about the analysis of substances, but also improving the existing analysis techniques and developing new ones.

Some of the common analysis methods are as follows:

- **Flame tests**: The test involves subjecting a given sample to the flame (reducing or oxidizing) and then observing the color of the flame. The color of the flame gives us an idea of a constituent present in the sample. This test is hardly used in industries or in a professional world.
- **Chemical tests**: It is used to identify functional groups in a given sample by conducting a series of chemical reaction on the sample.
- **Titrations (or Volumetric analysis)**: It involves the addition of a known titrant in the solution until the equivalence point is reached.
- **Gravimetry**: It is a quantitative technique that is used to estimate the amount of substance present based on the difference of mass after a change.
- **Chromatography**: It is a separation technique that consists of mobile phase (a fluid carrying a given sample) which flows on the stationary phase. Based on the affinity of the mobile phase ingredients towards the stationary phase, the retention of ingredients on the stationary phase takes place.
- **Spectroscopy**: It is the study of how atoms and molecules interact with electromagnetic radiations.
- **Electrochemical** analysis: It is a method of analysis in which the analyte is studied by passing electricity and measuring voltage and current over time.
- **Electrophoresis**: It is a separation method in which dispersed particles are separated under the influence of an electric field.

Importance of Analytical Chemistry

Analytical chemistry is the branch which is taught in almost all schools and colleges. But the applications of it are made in pharmaceutical industries, food factories, chemical industries, agricultural industries and in scientific laboratories. The tools used for this purpose are quite expensive which one cannot afford at home.

Applications of Analytical Chemistry

Some important applications of this branch of chemistry are listed below.

- The shelf lives of many medicines are determined with the help of analytical chemistry.
- It is used to check for the presence of adulterants in drugs.
- Soil can be tested to check for appropriate concentrations of minerals and nutrients that are necessary for plant growth.
- It is employed in the process of chromatography where the blood samples of a person are classified.

5.2. Physical Chemistry

As from the name Physical Chemistry is the combination of Physics and Chemistry. Physical Chemistry has a good overlap with some of the branches of Physics. It is a sub-branch of science that deals with the study of macroscopic properties like pressure, volume etc.; atomic properties like ionization energy, electronegativity, valency etc. It also deals with the structure of matter and energy.

Some of the areas of study in Physical Chemistry are mentioned below:

- **Chemical Kinetics**: It is the study of rates of chemical reaction.
- **Thermochemistry**: It is an area pertaining to thermodynamics which deals with heat in the chemical system and its relation to work.
- **Surface Chemistry**: It is an area of the study of chemical processes at surfaces of materials.
- **Photochemistry**: It is the study of chemical reactions which take place in the presence of light.
- **Spectroscopy**: It concerns with electromagnetic radiations and how they interact with atoms and molecules.

- **Statistical Mechanics**: It is the statistical study of large numbers of atom and molecules. Statistical Mechanics is one of a subject where Physics and Chemistry overlap each other.
- **Quantum Chemistry**: It is an application of Quantum Mechanics to the chemical system.
- **Electrochemistry**: It is a branch of physical chemistry which deals with chemical changes involving the movement of electrons between the electrodes.
- **Femtochemistry**: It is the study of chemical reactions in femtoscale (10−15 seconds). It helps us to understand each and every movement of molecules.

Applications of Physical Chemistry

Some applications of Physical chemistry are mentioned below

- A few physical chemists find employment in industries that are involved with the development of materials, including plastics, ceramics, catalysis, electronics, fuel formulation, batteries, surfactants and colloids, and personal care products, with most of them working as material scientists or analytical chemists.
- Physical chemistry requires significant mathematical and statistical understanding, and that combination is valuable in many industries that have large data sets that need to be mined for information. Wall Street financial firms, law firms, and venture capital firms are examples of places that hire scientists to read and analyze material from the chemical industry.
- Computational modeling is another application of physical chemistry and involves quantifying and predicting how materials will function. The pharmaceutical and materials industries especially conduct significant amounts of molecular modeling, but an advanced degree is usually required for this work.
- Many physical chemists work at national labs such as Lawrence Livermore National Laboratory, where they ensure the safety, security, and reliability of nuclear weapons, or Sandia National Laboratory, where they develop, engineer, and test the non-nuclear components of nuclear weapons.

5.3. Organic Chemistry

It is a branch of Chemistry which deals with the study of organic compounds. organic compounds are compounds which contain carbon-hydrogen bond. Carbon is capable of forming long C-C chains (called catenation). It is because of this property of carbon, it forms a tremendous number of compounds. This is a reason why organic compounds exceed inorganic compounds. Other than carbon and hydrogen, the elements widely found in organic compounds are oxygen, nitrogen, sulphur, phosphorus, and halogens (fluorine, chlorine and iodine). Organics compounds are used in agriculture, food, medicine, polymer, textile, insecticide, pharmaceutical, rubber, fuel, and consumer goods industries. Some of the industrial important organic chemicals are methane, ethylene, propylene, 1,2-dichloroethylene, methanol, isopropyl alcohol, butane, acetylene, polystyrene, glycerol, acetone, acetic acid, acetic anhydride, urea, toluene, phenol, aniline. glucose, fructose, starch etc.

Important areas in Organic Chemistry are mentioned below.

- **Polymer Chemistry**: It deals with the synthesis and properties of polymers.
- **Organometallics Chemistry**: It is the study of organometallic compounds which consist of compounds having a metal-carbon-hydrogen bond (organometallic bond). This field is included in both organic as well as inorganic chemistry.
- **Physical Organic Chemistry**: It is the study of reactivity and structure of organic chemicals.
- **Stereochemistry**: It is a chemistry that studies stereoisomers. It focusses on the spatial arrangement of atoms.
- **Medicinal Chemistry**: It involves the application of chemistry for medicine and drug development.
- **Bioorganic Chemistry**: It is the combination of Organic and Biochemistry.

Importance of Organic Chemistry

Organic chemistry is essential to understand the following concepts.

- Organic chemistry is a highly creative science in which chemists create new molecules and explore the properties of existing compounds.
- It is the most popular field of study for ACS chemists and Ph.D. chemists.
- Organic compounds are all around us. They are central to the economic growth of the United States in the rubber, plastics, fuel, pharmaceutical, cosmetics, detergent, coatings, dyestuff, and agrichemical industries, to name a few.
- The very foundations of biochemistry, biotechnology, and medicine are built on organic compounds and their role in life processes.
- Many modern, high-tech materials are at least partially composed of organic compounds.
- Organic chemists spend much of their time creating new compounds and developing better ways of synthesizing previously known compounds.

5.4. Inorganic Chemistry

It is a branch of Chemistry which deals with the study of inorganic compounds. Inorganic compounds are compounds which do not contain carbon-hydrogen bond. Inorganic compounds largely found beneath the earth surface: rocks and minerals, and others are produced in chemical industries. Inorganic chemicals have applications in paint, pigment, coating, fertilizer, surfactant, disinfectant, solar power industries. The largest inorganic chemicals produced in the world are sulphuric acid, hydrogen, nitrogen, ammonia, chlorine, phosphorus pentaoxide, nitric acid, hydrochloric acid, sodium hydroxide.

Some of the areas in Inorganic chemistry are as follows:

- **Coordination Chemistry**: It consists of the study of coordination complexes. Coordination complexes are composed of a center atom typically a metal surrounded by ligands or complexing agent.

- **Organometallic Chemistry**: It is the study of organometallic compounds which consist of compounds having a metal-carbon-hydrogen bond (organometallic bond). This field is included in both organic as well as inorganic chemistry.
- **Bioinorganic Chemistry**: This covers the interaction of inorganic species like metals in cells and tissues.
- **Solid-State Chemistry** (or Material Chemistry): It is the study of properties, structures of solid-state phase. It is a part of Solid-State Physics.

Applications of Inorganic Chemistry

Inorganic chemistry finds its high number of applications in various fields such as Biology, chemical, engineering, etc

- It is applied in the field of medicine and also in healthcare facilities.
- The most common application is the use of common salt or the compound Sodium hydroxide in our daily lives.
- Baking soda is used in the preparation of cakes and other foodstuffs.
- Many inorganic compounds are utilized in ceramic industries.
- In the electrical field, it is applied to the electric circuits as silicon in the computers, etc.
- Ammonia is used in the production of nylons, fibers, plastics, polyurethanes, hydrazine (used in jet and rocket fuels), and explosives.
- White powder pigment in paints, coatings, plastics, paper, inks, fibers, food, and cosmetics.

Importance of inorganic Chemistry

Catalysts, coatings, fuels, surfactants, fibers, superconductors, and drugs are researched and developed using inorganic chemistry. In inorganic chemistry important chemical reactions include double displacement reactions, acid-base reactions, and redox reactions.

5.5. Biochemistry

Biochemistry is the field of science that emphases on the study of chemical processes inside the biological system. Biochemistry is a new field compare to the above branches of chemistry. Professionals in this arena of Chemistry are called Biochemist. Biochemistry focusses on uses of chemistry to better understand biological systems like respiration, digestion, cellular metabolism etc. Biochemists work on diseases like cancer to develop better treatment; they also study molecular genetics to improve genes.

The important areas of study in Biochemistry are as follows:

- **Molecular Genetic**: It involves the studies of genes. It is closely related to genetic engineering.
- **Agricultural Biochemistry**: It focusses on the implementation of biochemistry to improve agriculture production.
- **Molecular Biochemistry**: It deals with the study of macromolecules like proteins, membranes, enzymes, nucleic acids, amino acids, viruses etc.
- **Clinical Biochemistry**: It is all about diseases and related topics.
- **Immunochemistry**: It is a branch of biochemistry that concerned with chemical reaction associated with the immune system.

Importance of Biochemistry

Biochemistry is essential to understand the following concepts.

- The chemical processes which transform diet into compounds that are characteristics of the cells of a particular species.
- The catalytic functions of enzymes.
- Utilizing the potential energy obtained from the oxidation of foodstuff consumed for the various energy-requiring processes of the living cell.
- The properties and structure of substances that constitute the framework of tissues and cells.
- To solve fundamental problems in medicine and biology.

6. Sub Branches of Chemistry

Here some of the Sub Branches of chemistry are discussed below.

1. Food Chemistry
2. Environmental Chemistry
3. Agricultural Chemistry
4. Industrial Chemistry
5. Polymer Chemistry
6. Pharmaceutical Chemistry
7. Geochemistry
8. Forensic Chemistry
9. Nuclear Chemistry
10. Chemical Engineering
11. Green Chemistry
12. Petrochemistry
13. Radiochemistry
14. Atmospheric Chemistry
15. Neurochemistry

6.1. Food Chemistry

Food science deals with the three biological parts of food

1. carbohydrates,
2. lipids
3. proteins.

Carbohydrates are sugars and starches, the chemical fuels required for our cells to operate.

Lipids are fats and oils and are essential components of cell membranes and to lubricate and cushion organs among the body. As a result of fats have a pair of.25 times the energy per gram than either carbohydrates or proteins, many folks try and limit their intake to avoid changing into overweight.

Proteins are complicated molecules composed of from a hundred to five hundred or additional amino acids that are in chains along and plicate into three-dimensional shapes necessary for the structure and performance of each cell. Our bodies will synthesize a number of the amino acids; but eight of them, the essential amino acids, should be taken in as a part of our food.

Food scientists are involved with the inorganic parts of food like its water content, minerals, vitamins and enzymes. Food chemists improve the standard, safety, storage and style of our food. Food chemists may go for personal trade to develop new merchandise or improve the process. They'll conjointly work for state agencies like the Food and Drug Administration to examine food merchandise and handlers to safeguard the U.S.A. from contamination or harmful practices. Food chemists take a look at the merchandise to provide data used for the nutrition labels or to work out however packaging and storage affect the security and quality of the food. Flavorists work chemically to vary the style of food. Chemists may additionally work on alternative ways that to boost sensory attractiveness, like enhancing color, odor or texture.

6.2. Environmental Chemistry

Environmental chemists study how chemicals act with the natural atmosphere. Environmental chemistry is a knowledge base study that involves each analytical chemistry and an understanding of bionomics. Environmental chemists should initially perceive the chemicals and chemical reactions gift in natural processes within the soil water and air. Sampling and analysis will then verify if human activities have contaminated the atmosphere or caused harmful reactions to have an effect on it.

Water quality is a very important space in environmental chemistry. "Pure" water doesn't exist in nature; it continually has some minerals or alternative substance dissolved in it. Water quality chemists take a look at rivers, lakes and ocean water for characteristics like dissolved element, salinity, turbidity, suspended sediments, and pH. Water destined for human consumption should be freed from harmful contaminants and will be treated with additives like halide and chemical elements to extend its safety.

6.3. Agricultural Chemistry

Agricultural chemistry is bothered with the substances and chemical reactions that are involved the assembly, protection and use of crops and stock. It's an extremely knowledge base field that depends on ties to several alternative sciences. Agricultural chemists may go with the Department of Agriculture, the Environmental Protection Agency, the Food and Drug Administration or for personal trade. Agricultural chemists develop fertilizers, pesticides and herbicides necessary for large-scale crop production. They have to conjointly monitor however these merchandises are used and their impacts on the atmosphere.

Agricultural biotechnology may be an invasive focus for several agricultural chemists. Genetically manipulating crops to be immune to the herbicides wont to management weeds within the fields needs elaborated understanding of each the plants and also the chemicals at the molecular level. Biochemists should perceive biological science, chemistry and business has to develop crops that are easier to move or that have an extended period of time.

6.4. Industrial Chemistry

The manufacture, sale, and distribution of chemical merchandise is one in all the cornerstones of a developed country. Chemists play a vital role within the manufacture, inspection, and safe handling of chemical merchandise, likewise as in development and general management. The manufacture of basic chemicals like chemical element, chlorine, ammonia, and oil of vitriol provides the raw materials for industries manufacturing textiles, agricultural merchandise, metals, paints, and pulp and paper. Specialty chemicals are created in smaller amounts for industries attached such merchandise as prescription drugs, foodstuffs, packaging, detergents, flavors, and fragrances. To an oversized extent, the industry takes the merchandise and reactions common to "bench-top" chemical processes and scales them up to industrial quantities.

The observance and management of bulk chemical processes, particularly with relevancy heat transfer, create issues typically tackled by chemists and chemical engineers. The disposal of by-products is also a significant downside for bulk chemical producers. These and different challenges of business chemistry set it excluding a lot of strictly intellectual disciplines of chemistry mentioned higher than. Yet, among the industry, there's a substantial quantity of elementary analysis undertaken among ancient specialties. Most giant chemical firms have research-and-development capability. Pharmaceutical corporations, for instance, operate giant analysis laboratories during which chemists check molecules for pharmacologic activity. The new merchandise and processes that are discovered in such laboratories are usually proprietary and become a supply of profit for the corporate funding the analysis. a good deal of the analysis conducted within the industry are often termed applied analysis as a result of its goals are closely tied to the merchandise and processes of the corporate involved. New technologies usually need a lot of chemical experience. The fabrication of, say, electronic microcircuits involves on the point of one hundred separate chemical steps from beginning to complete. Thus, the industry evolves with the technological advances of the fashionable world and at a constant time usually contributes to the speed of progress.

6.5. Polymer Chemistry

The simple substance ethene could be a gas composed of molecules with the formula CH_2CH_2. beneath bound conditions, several ethene molecules can be part of along to create a protracted chain known as polythene, with the formula $(CH_2CH_2)n$, wherever n could be a variable however sizable amount. polythene could be a robust, sturdy solid material quite totally different from ethene. it's Associate in Nursing example of a chemical compound, that could be a massive molecule created from several smaller molecules (monomers), sometimes joined along in an exceedingly linear fashion. several present substances, together with polyose, starch, cotton, wool, rubber, leather, proteins, and DNA, square measure polymers. polythene, nylon, and acrylics square measure samples of artificial polymers. The study of such materials lies at intervals the domain of chemical compound chemistry, a specialty that has flourished within the twentieth century. The investigation of natural polymers overlaps significantly with organic chemistry, however the synthesis of recent polymers, the investigation of chemical change processes, and therefore the characterization of the structure and properties of chemical compound materials all create distinctive issues for chemical compound chemists.

Polymer chemists have designed and synthesized polymers that adjust in hardness, flexibility, softening temperature, solubility in water, and biodegradability. They need created chemical compound materials that square measure as sturdy as steel nonetheless lighter and additional proof against corrosion. Oil, fossil fuel, and water pipelines square measure currently habitually made of plastic pipe. In recent years, automakers have enlarged their use of plastic parts to make lighter vehicles that consume less fuel. Alternative industries like those concerned within the manufacture of textiles, rubber, paper, and packaging materials square measure designed upon chemical compound chemistry.

Besides manufacturing new types of chemical compound materials, the researcher's square measure involved developing special catalysts that square measure needed by the large-scale industrial synthesis of economic polymers. While not such catalysts, the method change chemical action process would be slow inbound cases.

6.6. Pharmaceutical Chemistry

Pharmaceutical chemistry is concerned with the development and assessment of therapeutic compounds. Pharmaceutical chemistry encompasses drug style, drug synthesis, and also the analysis of drug effectuality (how effective it's in treating a condition) and drug safety. before the nineteenth century, colleges of pharmacy trained pharmacists and physicians the way to prepare medicative remedies from the natural organic product or inorganic materials. Flavorer medications and people remedies qualitative analysis back to ancient Egyptian, Greek, Roman, and Asian societies were administered with none information of their biological mechanism of action. it was not until the first 1800s that scientists began extracting chemicals from plants with putative therapeutic properties to isolate the active parts and establish them. By discovering and structurally characterizing compounds with meditative activity, chemist's square measure able to style new medication with increased efficiency and shriveled adverse facet effects.

Drug discovery is the core of pharmaceutical chemistry. The drug discovery method includes all the stages of drug development, from targeting a malady or medical condition to toxicity studies in animals, or even, by some definitions, testing the drug on human subjects. Typically, conditions that affect a bigger share of the population receive a lot of attention and a lot of analysis funding. Antiulcer medication and cholesterol-reducing agents square measure presently the therapeutic areas of greatest stress. To develop a drug to focus on a particular malady, researchers attempt to perceive the biological mechanism to blame for that condition. If the organic chemistry pathways leading up to the malady square measure understood, scientists conceive to style medication which will block one or many of the steps of the disease's progress. or else, a medication that boosts the body's own defense reaction is also acceptable.

6.7. **Geochemistry**

Geochemists mix chemistry and earth science to review the makeup and interaction between substances found within the Earth. Geochemists could pay longer in field studies than alternative styles of chemists. Several work for the U.S. earth science Survey or the Environmental Protection Agency in crucial however mining operations and waste will have an effect on water quality and also the atmosphere. they'll visit remote abandoned mines to gather samples and perform rough field evaluations, and so follow a stream through its watershed to gauge however contaminants are moving through the system. Crude oil geochemists are utilized by oil and gas firms to assist realize new energy reserves. They'll conjointly work on pipelines and oil rigs to forestall chemical reactions that might cause explosions or spills.

6.8. **Forensic Chemistry**

Forensic chemists capture and analyze the physical proof left behind at a criminal offense scene to assist verify the identities of the folks concerned furthermore on answer alternative important queries concerning however and why the crime was allotted. Rhetorical chemists use a large type of analyzation ways, like natural process, spectroscopic analysis and spectrometry.

In new analysis showing within the Journal of the yank Society of Mass spectroscopic analysis, scientists from the department of chemistry at American State University taken off to use optical device technology to the sphere of rhetorical science.

They developed a system that goes higher than and on the far side the identification of a fingerprint. The technique will capture molecules contained among a slur, together with lipids, proteins, genetic material, or maybe trace amounts of explosives, which may be more analyzed. The new tool basically takes the mystery out of characteristic the chemical composition of fingermarks at crime scenes.

The tool focuses an optical device — mistreatment mirrors and optical fibers — onto a surface containing a slur. The optical device then heats up any water or wetness on the surface, triggering chemical bonds within the water to stretch and vibrate, per the LSU faculty of Science web log. All of this targeted energy causes the water to "explode," turning it into a gas and separating biomolecules like DNA. This method is termed optical device ablation.

6.9. **Nuclear Chemistry**

Nuclear chemistry is the sub-field of chemistry dealing with radioactivity, nuclear processes, and transformations in the nuclei of atoms, such as nuclear transmutation and nuclear properties.

It is the chemistry of radioactive elements such as the actinides, radium and radon together with the chemistry associated with equipment (such as nuclear reactors) which are designed to perform nuclear processes. This includes the corrosion of surfaces and the behavior under conditions of both normal and abnormal operation (such as during an accident). An important area is the behavior of objects and materials after being placed into a nuclear waste storage or disposal site.

It includes the study of the chemical effects resulting from the absorption of radiation within living animals, plants, and other materials. The radiation chemistry controls much of radiation biology as radiation has an effect on living things at the molecular scale, to explain it another way the radiation alters the biochemicals within an organism, the alteration of the bio-molecules then changes the chemistry which occurs within the organism, this change in chemistry then can lead to a biological outcome. As a result, nuclear chemistry greatly assists the understanding of medical treatments (such as cancer radiotherapy) and has enabled these treatments to improve.

It includes the study of the production and use of radioactive sources for a range of processes. These include radiotherapy in medical applications; the use of radioactive tracers within industry, science and the environment; and the use of radiation to modify materials such as polymers.

It also includes the study and use of nuclear processes in non-radioactive areas of human activity. For instance, nuclear magnetic resonance (NMR) spectroscopy is commonly used in synthetic organic chemistry and physical chemistry and for structural analysis in macro-molecular chemistry.

Nuclear chemistry concerned with the study of nucleus, changes occurring in the nucleus, properties of the particles present in the nucleus and the emission or absorption of radiation from the nucleus

6.10. **Chemical Engineering**

Chemical engineers analyze and develop new materials or processes that involve chemical reactions. Chemical engineering combines a background in chemistry with engineering and economic science ideas to unravel technological issues. Chemical engineering jobs make up two main groups: industrial applications and development of recent merchandise.

Industries need chemical engineers to plan new ways that to form the producing of their merchandise easier and additional price effective. Chemical engineers are concerned in coming up with and in operation process plants, develop safety procedures for handling dangerous materials, and supervise the manufacture of nearly each product we have a tendency to use. Chemical engineers work to develop new merchandise and processes in each field from prescribed drugs to fuels and laptop parts.

6.11. Green Chemistry

Green Chemistry provides a unique forum for the publication of innovative research on the development of alternative green and sustainable technologies.

The scope of Green Chemistry is based on, but not limited to, the definition proposed by Anastas and Warner (Green Chemistry: Theory and Practice, P T Anastas and J C Warner, Oxford University Press, Oxford, 1998). Green chemistry is the utilization of a set of principles that reduces or eliminates the use or generation of hazardous substances in the design, manufacture and application of chemical products.

Green Chemistry is at the frontiers of this continuously-evolving interdisciplinary science and publishes research that attempts to reduce the environmental impact of the chemical enterprise by developing a technology base that is inherently non-toxic to living things and the environment. Submissions on all aspects of research relating to the endeavor are welcome.

The journal publishes original and significant cutting-edge research that is likely to be of wide general appeal. To be published, work must present a significant advance in green chemistry. Papers must contain a comparison with existing methods and demonstrate advantages over those methods before publication can be considered.

Coverage includes the following, but is not limited to:

Design: biomimicry, design for degradation/recycling/reduced toxicity

Reagents & Feedstocks: renewables, CO_2, solvents, auxiliary agents, waste utilization

Synthesis: organic, inorganic, catalysis, synthetic biology

Process: process design, intensification, separations, recycling, efficiency

Energy: renewable energy, fuels, photovoltaics, fuel cells, energy storage, energy carriers

Applications: electronics, dyes, consumer products, coatings, pharmaceuticals, preservatives, building materials, chemicals for industry/agriculture/mining

Impact: safety, metrics, LCA, sustainability, (eco) toxicology

Green chemistry is, by definition, a continuously-evolving frontier. Therefore, the inclusion of a particular material or technology does not, of itself, guarantee that a paper is suitable for the journal. To be suitable, the novel advance should have the potential for reduced environmental impact relative to the state of the art. Green Chemistry does not normally deal with research associated with 'end-of-pipe' or remediation issues.

6.12. **Petrochemistry**

The branch of Chemistry dealing with crude oil, petroleum, natural gas and its processing and refining. Petrochemistry is a very important segment since most of our energy requirements are fulfilled by end crude oil products like gasoline, diesel, LPG etc.

To understand the field of petrochemistry it's important to comprehend what petroleum is and where it comes from. Over millions of years, natural changes in organic materials have produced petroleum which has accumulated under the earth's surface. Petroleum rich areas are generally found in regions that support retention, such as porous sandstones.

Crude oils are naturally occurring liquids made up of various hydrocarbon compounds that differ in appearance and composition. Average composition rates are 84% carbon, 14% hydrogen, 1%-3% sulphur, and less than 1% each of nitrogen, oxygen, metals and salts. Depending on the sulphur content crude oils are either categorized as sweet or sour.

6.13. Radiochemistry

Radiochemistry is the chemistry of radioactive materials, where radioactive isotopes of elements are used to study the properties and chemical reactions of non-radioactive isotopes (often within radiochemistry the absence of radioactivity leads to a substance being described as being inactive as the isotopes are stable). Much of radiochemistry deals with the use of radioactivity to study ordinary chemical reactions. This is very different from radiation chemistry where the radiation levels are kept too low to influence the chemistry.

6.14. Atmospheric Chemistry

Atmospheric chemistry is a branch of atmospheric science in which the chemistry of the Earth's atmosphere and that of other planets is studied. It is a multidisciplinary approach of research and draws on environmental chemistry, physics, meteorology, computer modeling, oceanography, geology and volcanology and other disciplines. Research is increasingly connected with other areas of study such as climatology.

The composition and chemistry of the Earth's atmosphere is of importance for several reasons, but primarily because of the interactions between the atmosphere and living organisms. The composition of the Earth's atmosphere changes as result of natural processes such as volcano emissions, lightning and bombardment by solar particles from corona. It has also been changed by human activity and some of these changes are harmful to human health, crops and ecosystems. Examples of problems which have been addressed by atmospheric chemistry include acid rain, ozone depletion, photochemical smog, greenhouse gases and global warming. Atmospheric chemists seek to understand the causes of these problems, and by obtaining a theoretical understanding of them, allow possible solutions to be tested and the effects of changes in government policy evaluated.

6.15. Neurochemistry

Neurochemistry is the study of chemicals, including neurotransmitters and other molecules such as psychopharmaceuticals and neuropeptides, that control and influence the physiology of the nervous system. This field within neuroscience examines how neurochemicals influence the operation of neurons, synapses, and neural networks. Neurochemists analyze the biochemistry and molecular biology of organic compounds in the nervous system, and their roles in such neural processes including cortical plasticity, neurogenesis, and neural differentiation.

7. Introduction to Laboratory

A laboratory is a facility that provides controlled conditions in which scientific research, experiments and measurement of parameters are performed. Laboratory services are provided in a variety of settings: physician's offices, clinics, hospitals, and regional and national referral centers.

7.1. Laboratory Requirements

If you are setting up a new laboratory, evaluate the space to determine if it meets the requirements for handling the materials you intend to use. The use of hazardous materials requires the following:

Room Requirements

The laboratory space must have:

- Impervious and chemically resistant work surfaces;

- A sink; two sinks if you are using radioactive material;

- Safety shower (if hazardous chemicals are used);

- Eye-wash station (if hazardous chemicals and/or biological material is used);

- A fire extinguisher mounted to the wall or in an extinguisher cabinet;

- A functioning chemical fume hood for use of hazardous chemicals;

- A functioning biosafety cabinet for BL2;

- Chairs and furniture that are constructed of non-cloth material so that they can be effectively decontaminated;

- Electrical outlets sufficient in number and location to minimize the use of extension cords.

Laboratory Safety Management

- Handling hazardous materials requires a laboratory safety plan that identifies the hazards present and explains how to control them.

- Identify hazards in the laboratory space.

- Establish lab-specific training (e.g., conduct, PPE use) and emergency procedures (e.g., chemical spills, fire) for the lab.

- Establish Standard Operating Procedures (SOPs) for all hazardous procedures.

- Ensure that all training on SOPs, lab specific information, and emergency procedures is documented.

- Post emergency contact signs.

- Ensure that emergency equipment (e.g., fire extinguisher, spill kits, eyewash stations, and shower) is present.

- Establish correct waste disposal procedures.

Chemical Use

Before using chemicals, you must have to follow the following steps.

- Maintain a list of hazardous chemicals that includes chemical name, CAS#, location, hazard, and quantity.

- Provide access to Safety Data Sheets (SDS) for all chemicals.

- Establish and maintain appropriate chemical storage and segregation.

- Keep the amount of flammable liquids, flammable, oxidizing, and toxic compressed gases within the allowable limit.

7.2. Reagent Manufacturing Company

1. BDH (British Drug House), UK; Grade- Technical, GPR, AnalaR, Arister, Convol, Spectrosol etc.
2. Sigma-Aldrich, USA [ACS = American Chemical Society]
3. Merck, Germany
4. Fulka, Germany
5. RDH (Reidel De Hans), Germany
6. Loba, India

7.3. Reagent Labels

1. All solution labels meet all ISO, DOT and OSHA regulations and include the following information:
2. Expiration Date
3. Date of Manufacture
4. Standard Reference Material used
5. Actual Lot Analysis
6. Space for date received and date opened
7. NFPA diamond

7.4. Analytical Standard and CRMS

An analytical standard is a compound of suitable purity and known concentration to be used as a calibration standard for an assay. A certified reference material (CRM) is a material which has been certified by some trusted organization to be of a consistent quality and composition

- Certified Reference Materials (CRMs) are 'controls' or standards used to check the quality and metrological traceability of products, to validate analytical measurement methods, or for the calibration of instruments.

- A certified reference material is particular form of measurement standard.

A Certificate is issued for an SRM certified for one or more specific physical or engineering performance properties and may contain NIST reference, information, or both values in addition to certified values. ISO Guide 34:2000 – General requirements for the competence of reference material producers.

7.5. Lab Chemical Safety

DO

- Use the appropriate size container for the job.
- Get help when needed.
- Clean container after use with deionized water.
- Work under fume hood unless you have been told otherwise by the lab manger/supervisor.
- Use a funnel when pouring chemicals into a small container.
- Open bottles slowly to avoid spilling and allow vapors to escape.
- Know what type of reactions to expect.
- Eye protection: Chemicals, especially corrosive ones, and flying fragments of objects may cause serious damage. So, use of safety glasses is mandatory in laboratory work.
- Beware of hot glass: It cools very slowly and may be very hot without appearing so.
- Remember to triple- A(AAA): Always Add Acid to water.

DON'T

- Reuse container (adverse chemical reaction may occur).
- Eat, drink, smoke, or touch any body part before washing hands when working with chemicals.
- Be afraid to ask questions.
- Pour leftover chemicals back in its source container, contamination may result.
- Put your face close to the bottle when pouring.
- Puncture cap or lid of any bottle.

- Use any glass rod or tube without fire-polishing. Fire-polishing the sharp edges of glass rod or tube takes hardly few seconds, but saves you from injury which may occur in handling it.

- Insert any glass rod/tube into the cork without moistening the cork and the rod/tube.

- Point your test tube to neighbors or yourself, when heating substances in a test tube.

- Pour water into strong acid, the heat generated may break the container, always pour strong acid into water slowly and with constant stirring.

7.6. Maintenance of Work Environment

- At the end of the laboratory hour, leave your glassware clean & dry.
- Wipe out the desk top so that it does not get spotted and dirty.
- In course of work throw solids to the waste paper box, liquids into the sink.
- Never throw solid, filter paper and broken glass parts into the sink
- Never return unused chemicals to the stock bottles
- Always put the reagent bottles in their proper positions.
- Never insert your own pipettes or droppers into the stock solution.
- Always take a portion of the reagent in to a clean beaker/flash and from there you take with your pipettes/droppers.
- Do not lay down the stopper or a reagent bottle on the table. This may introduce impurities from the table top when you replace it.
- Do not heat graduated cylinders, bottles or burettes on a burner.

7.7. Quality

Quality can be defined as conformance to specifications. The degree to which a product meets the design specifications offering a satisfaction factor that fulfils all the expectations that a customer wants. Products are manufactured and controlled following normative regulations accepted in the market, so that in case of an inspection by a regulatory body, the product proves that it meets the requirements established by the related certifying organizations.

More specifically, in manufacturing, quality can be a measure of excellence or a state of being free from defects, deficiencies and significant variations. Quality is accomplished by a strict and consistent commitment to certain standards to achieve uniformity of a product in order to satisfy specific customer requirements. If an automobile company finds a defect in one of their cars and makes a product recall, customer reliability and therefore production will decrease because trust will be lost in the car's quality.

7.8. Quality Control (QC)

Quality control is the set of measures and procedures to follow in order to ensure that the quality of a product is maintained and improved against a set of benchmarks and that any errors encountered are either eliminated or reduced. The focus of quality control is to ensure that the product and product manufacturing are not only consistent but also in line with customer requirements.

Quality control is a part of quality assurance. One of the features of quality control is the use of well-defined controls. It brings standardization into the process. Most organizations have a quality control department that provides the set of standards to be followed for each product. Either an internal team or a third-party team is hired to determine whether the products that are delivered meet these standards. Quality control relies on testing of products, as product inspection gives a clearer picture of the quality of the end product. There are different standards available for quality control.

The quality of a product is often impacted by deviations from target standards and by the high variability around target specifications. Effective quality control should be able to address both these issues. Quality control can help businesses in improving their products in the market along with brand recognition. It also helps in addressing liability concerns, planning and decision making, and meeting customer needs. The effort and finance involved in product delivery can be much improved with the help of quality control.

7.9. Quality Assurance (QA)

Quality assurance (QA) is the process of verifying whether a product meets required specifications and customer expectations. QA is a process-driven approach that facilitates and defines goals regarding product design, development and production. QA's primary goal is tracking and resolving deficiencies prior to product release.

Organizations often designate separate QA departments, which increases customer confidence and credibility and improves efficiency and overall work processes.

Measurability is the key to QA. Products are tested and evaluated to determine whether they meet required performance specifications. QA may require many iterations and involve production delays.

An organization's QA approach generally emphasizes management, knowledge, skills, personal integrity, confidence, quality relationships and infrastructure.

If relevant expertise and skills are not present within an organization, consultants may be involved when new quality practices are introduced. Contracted experts employ a combination of procedural documentation with quality function deployment, capability maturity model integration and Six Sigma, etc.

7.10. **Research & Development (R&D)**

Research and development (R&D) include activities that companies undertake to innovate and introduce new products and services. It is often the first stage in the development process.

 R&D allows a company to stay ahead of its competition. Without an R&D program, a company may not survive on its own and may have to rely on other ways to innovate such as engaging in mergers and acquisitions (M&A) or partnerships. Through R&D, companies can design new products and improve their existing offerings.

R&D is separate from most operational activities performed by a corporation. The research and/or development is typically not performed with the expectation of immediate profit. Instead, it is expected to contribute to the long-term profitability of a company. R&D may lead to patents, copyrights, and trademarks as discoveries are made and products created.

7.11. **Sampling**

Sample: A portion of material collected according to a defined sampling procedure. The size of any sample should be sufficient to allow all anticipated test procedures to be carried out, including all reputation and samples.

Sampling: The process of taking a small portion from a lot/batch test and analysis.

Starting Materials Sampling Plan

When sampling starting materials, proper consideration has to be given to deciding on a sampling plan. The following are examples of sampling plans that could be used.

- **The "n plan":** The "n plan" should be used with great caution and only when the material to be sampled is considered uniform and is supplied from a recognized source.

- **The "p plan":** The "p plan" may be used when the material is uniform, is received from a recognized source and the main purpose is to test for identity.

- **The "r plan":** The "r plan" may be used when the material is suspected to be non-uniform and/or is received from a source that is not well known.

Packaging Materials Sampling Plan

Sampling plans for packaging materials should be based on defined sampling standards, from example, British Standard BS 6001-1, ISO 2859 or ANSI/ASQCZ 1.4-1993. The objective is to ensure that there is a low probability of accepting material that does not comply with the predefined acceptance level.

Finished Products Sampling Plan

As for packaging materials, sampling plans for finished products should be based on defined sampling, standards such as BS 6001-1, ISO 2859 or ANSI/ASQCZ 1.4-1993. In some cases, it may be sufficient to limit examination of finished goods to visual inspection only.

7.12. Accuracy & Precision

Accuracy refers to the closeness of a measured value to a standard or known value. For example, if in lab you obtain a weight measurement of 3.2 kg for a given substance, but the actual or known weight is 10 kg, then your measurement is not accurate. In this case, your measurement is not close to the known value.

Precision refers to the closeness of two or more measurements to each other. Using the example above, if you weigh a given substance five times, and get 3.2 kg each time, then your measurement is very precise. Precision is independent of accuracy. You can be very precise but inaccurate, as described above. You can also be accurate but imprecise.

For example, if on average, your measurements for a given substance are close to the known value, but the measurements are far from each other, then you have accuracy without precision.

A good analogy for understanding accuracy and precision is to imagine a basketball player shooting baskets. If the player shoots with accuracy, his aim will always take the ball close to or into the basket. If the player shoots with precision, his aim will always take the ball to the same location which may or may not be close to the basket. A good player will be both accurate and precise by shooting the ball the same way each time and each time making it in the basket.

7.13. Methods

Normally for performing chemical analysis a chemist has to follow different written methods approved from reliable organizations.

- Standard methods from American Society for Testing Materials (ASTM), Food and Drug Administration (FDA)
- Non-Standard methods from personal research
- In-house methods from Government or Private research organizations

7.14. International Organization for Standardization (ISO)

ISO (International Organization for Standardization) is a non-governmental organization that forms a bridge between the public and private sectors and is the largest standards organization in the world. It is a network of standards institutes from 164 countries with a central office in Geneva, Switzerland, that coordinates the system.

Many of its member institutes are part of the governmental structure of their countries or are mandated by their government. Some members have their roots uniquely in the private sector, having been set up by national partnerships of industry associations.

Therefore, ISO enables a consensus to be reached on solutions that meet both the requirements of business and the broader needs of society.

ISO-17025:2017

ISO/IEC 17025:2017 for General requirements for the competence of testing and calibration laboratories ISO/IEC 17025:2017 specifies the general requirements for the competence, impartiality and consistent operation of laboratories.

It is applicable to all organizations performing laboratory activities, regardless of the number of personnel.

Laboratory customers, regulatory authorities, organizations and schemes using peer-assessment, accreditation bodies, and others use ISO/IEC 17025:2017 in confirming or recognizing the competence of laboratories.

ISO-14001:2015

ISO 14001:2015 for Environmental management systems. ISO 14001:2015 specifies the requirements for an environmental management system that an organization can use to enhance its environmental performance. ISO 14001:2015 is intended for use by an organization seeking to manage its environmental responsibilities in a systematic manner that contributes to the environmental pillar of sustainability.

ISO 14001:2015 helps an organization achieve the intended outcomes of its environmental management system, which provide value for the environment, the organization itself and interested parties. Consistent with the organization's environmental policy, the intended outcomes of an environmental management system include: enhancement of environmental performance; fulfilment of compliance obligations; achievement of environmental objectives.

ISO-9001:2015

ISO 9001:2015 for Quality management systems. ISO 9001:2015 specifies requirements for a quality management system when an organization:

a) needs to demonstrate its ability to consistently provide products and services that meet customer and applicable statutory and regulatory requirements, and

b) aims to enhance customer satisfaction through the effective application of the system, including processes for improvement of the system and the assurance of conformity to customer and applicable statutory and regulatory requirements.

All the requirements of ISO 9001:2015 are generic and are intended to be applicable to any organization, regardless of its type or size, or the products and services it provides.

ISO-22000

ISO 22000 for Food safety management. Whatever their size, or product, all food producers have a responsibility to manage the safety of their products and the well-being of their consumers. That's why ISO 22000 exists.

The consequences of unsafe food can be serious. ISO's food safety management standards help organizations identify and control food safety hazards, at the same time as working together with other ISO management standards, such as ISO 9001. Applicable to all types of producer, ISO 22000 provides a layer of reassurance within the global food supply chain, helping products cross borders and bringing people food that they can trust.

7.15. Good manufacturing Practice (GMP)

Good manufacturing practice (GMP) is a system for ensuring that products are consistently produced and controlled according to quality standards. It is designed to minimize the risks involved in any pharmaceutical production that cannot be eliminated through testing the final product.

GMP covers all aspects of production; from the starting materials, premises and equipment to the training and personal hygiene of staff. Detailed, written procedures are essential for each process that could affect the quality of the finished product. There must be systems to provide documented proof that correct procedures are consistently followed at each step in the manufacturing process - every time a product is made.

GMP is necessary if there is a quality control laboratory. Good quality must be built in during the manufacturing process; it cannot be tested into the product afterwards. GMP prevents errors that cannot be eliminated through quality control of the finished product. Without GMP it is impossible to be sure that every unit of a medicine is of the same quality as the units of medicine tested in the laboratory

7.16. Standard Operating Procedure (SOP)

It is a set of step-by-step instructions compiled by an organization to help workers carry out complex routine operations. SOPs aim to achieve efficiency, quality output and uniformity of performance, while reducing miscommunication and failure to comply with industry regulations.

An SOP, in fact, defines expected practices in all industry where quality standards exist. SOPs play an important role in your small business. It is a part of quality assurance. SOPs are policies, procedures and standards you need in the operations, marketing and administration disciplines within your business to ensure success. These can create:

- efficiencies, and therefore profitability
- consistency and reliability in production and service
- fewer errors in all areas
- a way to resolve conflicts between partners
- a healthy and safe environment
- protection of employers in areas of potential liability and personnel matters
- a roadmap for how to resolve issues – and the removal of emotion from troubleshooting – allowing needed focus on solving the problem
- a first line of defense in any inspection, whether it be by a regulatory body, a partner or potential partner, a client, or a firm conducting due diligence for a possible purchase
- value added to industry.

8. Fundamentals of Chemical Analysis

8.1. Standardization

Standardization is the process of determining the exact concentration (molarity) of a solution. Titration is one type of analytical procedure often used in standardization. Here an exact volume of unknown substance is reacted with a known amount of another substance mostly primary standard substances.

Example of standardization: The molarity of a sodium hydroxide solution (NaOH) can be determined by titrating a sample of potassium acid phthalate (KHP; $HKC_8H_4O_4$) with the NaOH. In the second procedure the standardized NaOH can be used to determine the molarity of a hydrochloric solution (HCl).

8.2. Calibration

In chemistry, calibration is defined as the act of making sure that a scientific process or instrument will produce results which are accurate. In more complex terms, calibration is the act which determines the functional relationship between measured values and analytical quantities.

Any instrument used in research needs to be properly calibrated to make sure the data it produces is valid and can be used by others. Over time, instruments can 'drift' due to normal wear and tear and can, therefore, give inaccurate results – this is why it's important that machines are properly calibrated before use. Any instrument used in scientific research needs to be properly calibrated before it is used – this is done through adjustment of the precision and accuracy of the instruments

There are two main ways of calibrating an instrument

1. The working curve method
2. The standard addition method.

8.3. Validation

Method validation is a key element in the establishment of reference methods and within the assessment of a laboratory's competence in generating dependable analytical records. Validation has been placed within the context of the procedure, generating chemical data. Analytical method validation, thinking about the maximum relevant processes for checking the best parameters of analytical methods, using numerous relevant overall performance indicators inclusive of selectivity, specificity, accuracy, precision, linearity, range, limit of detection (LOD), limit of quantification (LOQ), ruggedness, and robustness are severely discussed in an effort to prevent their misguided utilization and ensure scientific correctness and consistency among publications.

Analytical method validation is an essential requirement to perform the chemical evaluation. Method validation is a procedure of performing numerous assessments designed to verify that an analytical test system is suitable for its intended reason and is capable of providing beneficial and legitimate analytical data. A validation examine includes testing multiple attributes of a method to determine that it may provide useful and valid facts whilst used robotically. To accurately investigate method parameters, the validation test ought to consist of normal test conditions, which includes product excipients. Therefore, a method validation examine is product-specific.

8.4. Units

There is international agreement that the units used for physical quantities in science and technology should be those of the International System of Units, or SI. The Physical Chemistry Division of the International Union of Pure and Applied Chemistry, or IUPAC, produces a manual of recommended symbols and terminology for physical quantities and units based on the SI.

Table 1.1 SI base units

Physical quantity	SI unit	Symbol
length	meter[a]	m
mass	kilogram	kg
time	second	s
thermodynamic temperature	kelvin	K
amount of substance	mole	mol
electric current	ampere	A
luminous intensity	candela	cd

[a]or metre

The SI is built on the seven base units listed in Table 1.1. These base units are independent physical quantities that are sufficient to describe all other physical quantities.

Table 1.2 SI derived units

Physical quantity	Unit	Symbol	Definition of unit
force	newton	N	$1\,N = 1\,m\,kg\,s^{-2}$
pressure	pascal	Pa	$1\,Pa = 1\,N\,m^{-2} = 1\,kg\,m^{-1}\,s^{-2}$
Celsius temperature	degree Celsius	°C	$t/°C = T/K - 273.15$
energy	joule	J	$1\,J = 1\,N\,m = 1\,m^2\,kg\,s^{-2}$
power	watt	W	$1\,W = 1\,J\,s^{-1} = 1\,m^2\,kg\,s^{-3}$
frequency	hertz	Hz	$1\,Hz = 1\,s^{-1}$
electric charge	coulomb	C	$1\,C = 1\,A\,s$
electric potential	volt	V	$1\,V = 1\,J\,C^{-1} = 1\,m^2\,kg\,s^{-3}\,A^{-1}$
electric resistance	ohm	Ω	$1\,\Omega = 1\,V\,A^{-1} = 1\,m^2\,kg\,s^{-3}\,A^{-2}$

Table 1.2 lists derived units for some additional physical quantities used in thermodynamics. The derived units have exact definitions in terms of SI base units, as given in the last column of the table.

Table 1.3 Non-SI derived units

Physical quantity	Unit	Symbol	Definition of unit
volume	liter[a]	L[b]	$1\,L = 1\,dm^3 = 10^{-3}\,m^3$
pressure	bar	bar	$1\,bar = 10^5\,Pa$
pressure	atmosphere	atm	$1\,atm = 101{,}325\,Pa = 1.01325\,bar$
pressure	torr	Torr	$1\,Torr = (1/760)\,atm = (101{,}325/760)\,Pa$
energy	calorie[c]	cal[d]	$1\,cal = 4.184\,J$

[a] or litre   [b] or l   [c] or thermochemical calorie   [d] or cal_{th}

The units listed in Table 1.3 are sometimes used in thermodynamics but are not part of the SI. They do, however, have exact definitions in terms of SI units and so offer no problems of numerical conversion to or from SI units.

Table 1.4 SI prefixes

Fraction	Prefix	Symbol		Multiple	Prefix	Symbol
10^{-1}	deci	d		10	deka	da
10^{-2}	centi	c		10^2	hecto	h
10^{-3}	milli	m		10^3	kilo	k
10^{-6}	micro	μ		10^6	mega	M
10^{-9}	nano	n		10^9	giga	G
10^{-12}	pico	p		10^{12}	tera	T
10^{-15}	femto	f		10^{15}	peta	P
10^{-18}	atto	a		10^{18}	exa	E
10^{-21}	zepto	z		10^{21}	zetta	Z
10^{-24}	yocto	y		10^{24}	yotta	Y

Any of the symbols for units listed in Tables 1.1–1.3, except kg and °C, may be preceded by one of the prefix symbols of Table 1.4 to construct a decimal fraction or multiple of the unit. (The symbol g

65

may be preceded by a prefix symbol to construct a fraction or multiple of the gram.) The combination of prefix symbol and unit symbol is taken as a new symbol that can be raised to a power without using parentheses, as in the following examples:

$$1mg=1\times10^{-3}g \quad 1mg=1\times10^{-3}g$$

$$1cm=1\times10^{-2}m \quad 1cm=1\times10^{-2}m$$

$$1cm^3=(1\times10^{-2}m)^3=1\times10^{-6}m^3$$

$$1cm^3=(1\times10^{-2}m)^3=1\times10^{-6}m^3$$

Amount of substance and amount

The physical quantity formally called amount of substance is a counting quantity for particles, such as atoms or molecules, or for other chemical entities. The counting unit is invariably the mole, defined as the amount of substance containing as many particles as the number of atoms in exactly 12 grams of pure carbon-12 nuclide, ^{12}C. One mole of H_2O molecules, for example, has a mass of 18.0153 grams (where 18.0153 is the relative molecular mass of H_2O) and contains 6.02214×10^{23} molecules (where $6.02214\times10^{23}mol^{-1}$ is the Avogadro constant to six significant digits). The same statement can be made for any other substance if 18.0153 is replaced by the appropriate atomic mass or molecular mass value.

The symbol for amount of substance is n. It is admittedly awkward to refer to $n(H_2O)$ as "the amount of substance of water." This book simply shortens "amount of substance" to amount. An alternative name suggested for n is "chemical amount." Thus, "the amount of water in the system" refers not to the mass or volume of water, but to the number of H_2O molecules in the system expressed in a counting unit such as the mole.

8.5. Solution Strength

8.5.1.   % of Solution

One way to describe the concentration of a solution is by the percent of a solute in the solvent. The percent can further be determined in one of two ways: (1) the ratio of the mass of the solute divided by the mass of the solution or (2) the ratio of the volume of the solute divided by the volume of the solution.

Mass Percent

When the solute in a solution is a solid, a convenient way to express the concentration is a mass percent, $\left(\frac{mass}{mass}\right)$ which is the grams of solute per 100 g of solution.

$$\text{Percent by mass} = \frac{\text{mass of solute}}{\text{mass of solution}} \times 100\%$$

Suppose that a solution was prepared by dissolving 25.0 g of sugar into 100 g of water. The percent by mass would be calculated by:

$$\text{Percent by mass} = \frac{25 \text{ g sugar}}{125 \text{ g solution}} \times 100\% = 20\% \text{ sugar}$$

Sometimes you may want to make up a particular mass of solution of a given percent by mass and need to calculate what mass of the solvent to use. For example, you need to make 3000 g of a 5% solution of sodium chloride. You can rearrange and solve for the mass of solute.

$$\text{mass of solute} = \frac{\text{percent by mass}}{100\%} \times \text{mass of solution} = \frac{5\%}{100\%} \times 3000 \text{ g} = 150 \text{ g NaCl}$$

You would need to weigh out 150 g of NaCl and add it to 2850 g of water. Notice that it was necessary to subtract the mass of the NaCl (150 g) from the mass of solution (3000 g) to calculate the mass of the water that would need to be added.

Volume Percent

The percentage of solute in a solution can more easily be determined by volume when the solute and solvent are both liquids. The volume of the solute divided by the volume of solution expressed as a percent

$$\text{Percent by volume} = \frac{\text{volume of solute}}{\text{volume of solution}} \times 100\%$$

$$= \frac{40 \text{ mL ethanol}}{240 \text{ mL solution}} \times 100\%$$

$$= 16.7\% \text{ ethanol}$$

yields the percent by volume $\left(\frac{\text{volume}}{\text{volume}}\right)$ of the solution. If a solution is made by adding 40 mL of ethanol to 20 mL of water, the percent by volume is:

8.5.2.   Parts Per Million (ppm)

Parts Per Million (ppm) is a measurement of the concentration of a solution. For very dilute solutions, weight/weight (w/w) and weight/volume (w/v) concentrations are sometimes expressed in parts per million.

1 ppm is one part by weight, or volume, of solute in 1 million parts by weight, or volume, of solution.

In weight/volume (w/v) terms,

$$1 \text{ ppm} = 1\text{g m}^{-3} = 1 \text{ mg L}^{-1} = 1 \text{ }\mu\text{g mL}^{-1}$$

In weight/weight (w/w) terms,

$$1 \text{ ppm} = 1 \text{ mg kg}^{-1} = 1 \text{ }\mu\text{g g}^{-1}$$

ppm is an abbreviation of parts per million. ppm is a value that represents the part of a whole number in units of 1/1000000.

One ppm is equal to 1/1000000 of the whole:

$1\text{ppm} = 1/1000000 = 0.000001 = 1\times10^{-6}$

One ppm is equal to 0.0001%:

$1\text{ppm} = 0.0001\%$

Concentration in ppm

The concentration C in ppm is also equal to the solute mass m_{solute} in milligrams (mg) divided by the solution mass $m_{solution}$ in kilograms (kg):

$$C_{(ppm)} = m_{solute}\ (mg) / m_{solution}\ (kg)$$

When the solution is water, the volume of mass of one kilogram is approximately one liter.

The concentration C in ppm is also equal to the solute mass m_{solute} in milligrams (mg) divided by the water solution volume $V_{solution}$ in liters (L):

$$C_{(ppm)} = m_{solute}\ (mg) / V_{solution}\ (L)$$

Percentage to ppm

The part P in ppm is equal to the part P in percent (%) times 10000:

$$P(ppm) = P(\%) \times 10000$$

Example

Find how many ppm are in 6%:

$$P(ppm) = 6\% \times 10000 = 60000\text{ppm}$$

8.5.3.   Parts Per Billion (ppb)

A weight to weight ratio used to describe concentrations. Parts per billion (ppb) is the number of units of mass of a contaminant per 1000 million units of total mass.

Also µg/L or micrograms per liter.

$1ppb = 1/1000000000 = 0.000000001 = 1 \times 10^{-9}$

ppb is used to measure the concentration of a contaminant in soils and sediments. In that case 1 ppb equals 1 µg of substance per kg of solid (µg/kg).

ppb is also sometimes used to describe small concentrations in water, in which case 1 ppb is equivalent to 1 µg/l because a liter of water weighs approximately a 1000 000 µg. This use of ppb tends to be phased out in favour of µg/l.

ppb is often used to describe concentrations of contaminants in air (as a volume fraction). In this case the conversion of ppb to µg/m3 depends on the molecular weight of the contaminant.

For example, 1 ppb chlorine represents one part of chlorine in one thousand million parts of air by weight, which is 1.45 µg/m3.

8.5.4.   Molarity

Molarity (M) is defined as the number of moles of solute per liter of solution. The units of molarity are M or mol/L. A 1 M solution is said to be "one molar."

Molarity = moles of solute/liters of solution

Mole = mass / molecular mass

Suppose we have to prepare 10 g 500 ml NaCl solution.

Here mass of NaCl is 10g

Molecular mass of NaCl is 58.5

Volume = 500ml = 0.5 L

So the molarity is = mole / molecular mass

$$= (mass / molecular\ mass) / volume$$

$$= (10/58.5) / 0.5\ molL^{-1}$$

$$= 0.342\ M$$

To convert percentage into molarity

$$\ldots\ldots\ldots\ldots\ldots\ldots\ldots\ldots\ldots\ldots\ldots = (\% * 1000) / (molecular\ mass * 100)$$

To convert ppm into molarity

$$\ldots\ldots\ldots\ldots\ldots\ldots\ldots\ldots\ldots = (ppm * 1000) / (molecular\ mass * 10^6)$$

8.5.5. Normality

Normality in chemistry is one of the expressions used to measure the concentration of a solution. It is abbreviated as 'N' and is sometimes referred to as the equivalent concentration of a solution. It is mainly used as a measure of reactive species in a solution and during titration reactions or particularly in situations involving acid-base chemistry.

Normality is described as the number of gram or mole equivalents of solute present in one liter of a solution. When we say equivalent, it is the number of moles of reactive units in a compound.

Normality = Number of gram equivalents × [volume of solution in liter]$^{-1}$

Number of gram equivalents = weight of solute × [Equivalent weight of solute]$^{-1}$

Equivalent weight = mass / equivalence number

So normality is

N = Weight of Solute (gram) × [Equivalent weight × Volume (L)]

The relationship between molarity and normality

Normality and molarity are two important and commonly used expressions in chemistry. They are used to indicate the quantitative measurement of a substance

Normality = Molarity * equivalence number

8.5.6.   Molality

Molality (m), or molal concentration, is the amount of a substance dissolved in a certain mass of solvent. It is defined as the moles of a solute per kilograms of a solvent. The units of molality are m or mol/kg.

Molality, m = moles solute / kilograms solvent

Since the volume of a solution is dependent on ambient temperature and pressure, mass can be more relevant for measuring solutions. In these cases, molality (not molarity) is the appropriate measurement.

8.5.7.   Solubility

The maximum amount of solute that can dissolve in a known quantity of solvent at a certain temperature is its solubility.

A solution is a homogeneous mixture of one or more solutes in a solvent. Sugar cubes added to a cup of tea or coffee is a common example of a solution. The property which helps sugar molecules to dissolve is known as solubility.

Hence, the term solubility can be defined as a property of a substance (solute) to dissolve in a given solvent. A solute is any substance which can be either solid or liquid or gas dissolved in a solvent.

Solubility has three types

   I.   Liquids In Liquids
  II.   Solids In Liquids
 III.   Gases In Liquids

Factors Affecting Solubility:

The solubility of a substance depends on the physical and chemical properties of that substance. In addition to this, there are a few conditions which can manipulate it. Temperature, pressure and the type of bond and forces between the particles are few among them.

Temperature:

By changing the temperature, we can increase the soluble property of a solute. Generally, water dissolves solutes at 20° C or 100° C. Sparingly soluble solid or liquid substances can be dissolved completely by increasing the temperature. But in the case of gaseous substance, temperature inversely influences solubility i.e. as the temperature increases gases expand and escapes from their solvent.

Forces and Bonds:

Like dissolves in like. The type of intermolecular forces and bonds vary among each molecule. The chances of solubility between two unlike substances are more challengeable than the like substances. For example, water is a polar solvent where a polar solute like ethanol is easily soluble.

Pressure:

Gaseous substances are much influenced than solids and liquids by pressure. When the partial pressure of gas increases, the chance of its solubility is also increased. A soda bottle is an example of where CO_2 is bottled under high pressure.

8.5.8.   pH of Solution

pH is defined as the measure of hydrogen ion concentration which is used for measuring the acidity or alkalinity of a given solution.

Following is the equation that is used for calculating the pH:

$pH = -\log[H+]$

Values of pH

The range of the pH scale varies from 0 to 14. Solutions having a value of pH ranging 0 to 7 on pH scale are known as acidic and for the value of pH ranging 7 to 14 on pH scale are called basic solutions. Solutions having the value of pH equal to 7 on pH scale are termed as neutral solutions.

The pH scale is logarithmic and as a result, each whole pH value below 7 is ten times more acidic than the next higher value. For example, pH 4 is ten times more acidic than pH 5 and 100 times (10 times 10) more acidic than pH 6. The same holds true for pH values above 7, each of which is ten times more alkaline (another way to say basic) than the next lower whole value. For example, pH 10 is ten times more alkaline than pH 9 and 100 times (10 times 10) more alkaline than pH 8.

8.5.9.   Buffer Solution

The buffer solution is a solution able to maintain its Hydrogen ion concentration (pH) with only minor changes on the dilution or addition of a small amount of either acid or base. Buffer Solutions are used in fermentation, food preservatives, drug delivery, electroplating, printing, the activity of enzymes, blood oxygen carrying capacity need specific hydrogen ion concentration (pH).

Solutions of a weak acid and its conjugate base or weak base and its conjugate acid are able to maintain pH and are buffer solutions.

Types of Buffer Solution

The two primary types into which buffer solutions are broadly classified into are acidic and alkaline buffers.

Acidic Buffers

As the name suggests, these solutions are used to maintain acidic environments. Acid buffer has acidic pH and is prepared by mixing a weak acid and its salt with a strong base. An aqueous solution of an equal concentration of acetic acid and sodium acetate has a pH of 4.74. pH of these solutions is below seven

These solutions consist of a weak acid and a salt of a weak acid. An example of an acidic buffer solution is a mixture of sodium acetate and acetic acid (pH = 4.75).

Alkaline Buffers

These buffer solutions are used to maintain basic conditions. Basic buffer has a basic pH and is prepared by mixing a weak base and its salt with strong acid. The aqueous solution of an equal concentration of ammonium hydroxide and ammonium chloride has a pH of 9.25. The pH of these solutions is above seven

They contain a weak base and a salt of the weak base. An example of an alkaline buffer solution is a mixture of ammonium hydroxide and ammonium chloride (pH = 9.25).

8.6. Water Quality Parameters

8.6.1.   DO

Dissolved oxygen (DO) is a measure of how much oxygen is dissolved in the water - the amount of oxygen available to living aquatic organisms. The amount of dissolved oxygen in a stream or lake can tell us a lot about its water quality.

Oxygen enters the water by direct absorption from the atmosphere, by rapid movement, or as a waste product of plant photosynthesis. Water temperature and the volume of moving water can affect dissolved oxygen levels. Oxygen dissolves easier in cooler water than warmer water.

Adequate dissolved oxygen is important for good water quality and necessary to all forms of life. Dissolved oxygen levels that drop below 5.0 mg/L cause stress to aquatic life. Lower concentrations cause greater stress. Oxygen levels that go below 1-2 mg/L for a few hours may result in large fish kills. Healthy water should generally have dissolved oxygen concentrations above 6.5-8 mg/L and between about 80-120 %.

Dissolved oxygen is best measured directly in the water using a calibrated dissolved oxygen sensor. This sensor can measure the amount of dissolved oxygen directly in the water as mg/L or as a percent dissolved oxygen (%DO).

8.6.2.   BOD

Biochemical oxygen demand, or BOD, is a chemical procedure for determining the amount of dissolved oxygen needed by aerobic biological organisms in a body of water to break down organic material present in a given water sample at certain temperature over a specific time period.

Biochemical oxygen demand directly affects the amount of dissolved oxygen in rivers and streams. The rate of oxygen consumption is affected by a number of variables: temperature, pH, the presence of certain kinds of microorganisms, and the type of organic and inorganic material in the water.

The greater the value, the more rapidly oxygen is depleted in the stream. This means less oxygen is available to higher forms of aquatic life. The consequences of high BOD are the same as those for low dissolved oxygen: aquatic organisms become stressed, suffocate, and die.

Biochemical oxygen demand is affected by the same factors that affect dissolved oxygen. Measuring biochemical oxygen demand requires taking two measurements. One is measured immediately for dissolved oxygen (initial), and the second is incubated in the lab for 5 days and then tested for the amount of dissolved oxygen remaining (final). This represents the amount of oxygen consumed by microorganisms to break down the organic matter present in the sample during the incubation period. It is not a precise quantitative test, although it is widely used as an indication of the organic quality of water. It is most commonly expressed in milligrams of oxygen consumed per liter of sample during 5 days (BOD_5) of incubation at 20°C and is often used as a robust surrogate of the degree of organic pollution of water

8.6.3.   COD

COD refers to the chemical oxygen demand, which measures the amount of DO, required by the decomposition of organic matter and the oxidation of inorganic chemicals like ammonia and nitrite. COD measurements are commonly made with the samples of wastewater or natural water, which are contaminated by domestic and industrial wastes.

The COD is often measured using a strong oxidant (e.g. potassium dichromate, potassium iodate, potassium permanganate) under acidic conditions. A known excess amount of the oxidant is added to the sample. Once oxidation is complete, the concentration of organics in the sample is calculated by measuring the amount of oxidant remaining in the solution. This is usually done by titration, using an indicator solution. COD is expressed in mg/L, which indicates the mass of oxygen consumed per liter of solution.

The COD test only requires 2-3 hours, while the Biochemical (or Biological) Oxygen Demand (BOD) test requires 5 days. It measures all organic contaminants, including those that are not biodegradable. There is a relationship between BOD and COD for each specific sample, but it must be established empirically. COD test results can then be used to estimate the BOD of a given sample. Unlike for the BOD test, toxic compounds (such as heavy metals and cyanides) in the samples to be analyzed do not have an effect on the oxidants used in the COD test. Therefore, the COD test can be used to measure the strength of wastes that are too toxic for the BOD test. Some organic molecules (e.g., benzene, pyridine) are relatively resistant to dichromate oxidation and may give a falsely low COD.

8.6.4.   Hardness

The simple definition of water hardness is the amount of salts of calcium and magnesium principally as bicarbonates, chlorides, and sulfates. Ferrous iron may also be present; oxidized to the ferric form, it appears as a reddish-brown stain on washed fabrics and enameled surfaces.

Types of Hardness of Water

The hardness of water can be classified into two types:

1. Temporary Hardness
2. Permanent Hardness

Temporary Hardness of Water:

The presence of magnesium and calcium carbonates in water makes it temporarily hard. In this case, the hardness in water can be removed by boiling the water.

When we boil water the soluble salts of $Mg(HCO_3)_2$ is converted to $Mg(OH)_2$ which is insoluble and hence gets precipitated and is removed. After filtration, the water we get is soft water.

Permanent Hardness of Water:

When the soluble salts of magnesium and calcium are present in the form of chlorides and sulfides in water, we call it permanent hardness because this hardness cannot be removed by boiling.

We can remove this hardness by treating the water with washing soda. Insoluble carbonates are formed when washing soda reacts with the sulfide and chloride salts of magnesium and calcium and thus hard water is converted to soft water.

Total hardness

Total hardness corresponds to the sum of the permanent and the temporary hardness. Because it is the precise mixture of minerals dissolved in the water, together with the water's pH and temperature, that determines the behavior of the hardness, a single-number scale does not adequately describe hardness.

8.6.5.   Turbidity

Turbidity is caused by particles suspended or dissolved in water that scatter light making the water appear cloudy or murky. It is a measure of the degree to which the water loses its transparency due to the presence of suspended particulates.

The more total suspended solids in the water, the murkier it seems and the higher the turbidity. Particulate matter can include sediment - especially clay and silt, fine organic and inorganic matter, soluble colored organic compounds, algae, and other microscopic organisms.

Turbidity is measured using specialized optical equipment in a laboratory or in the field. A light is directed through a water sample, and the amount of light scattered is measured. The unit of measurement is called a Nephelometric Turbidity Unit (NTU), which comes in several variations. The greater the scattering of light, the higher the turbidity. Low turbidity values indicate high water clarity; high values indicate low water clarity.

8.6.6.   Conductivity

Conductivity is nothing but the measure of the capability of water to pass the flow of electric current. This ability of conductance is said to be directly proportional to the concentration of the ions present in the water.

The Compounds which dissolve into the ions are known as the electrolytes. The more the number of ions present in the electrolyte, then the higher is the conductivity of water. In a similar way, fewer the number of ions present in water, then less conductive is the conductivity of water. De-ionized or distilled water can also act as an insulator due to the very low value of conductivity. Seawater is said to possess a very high value of conductivity.

Pure water is said to be a bad conductor of electricity. Normal water is said to have impurities present in the form of ions called minerals etc. These ions are known to be responsible for the conduction of electric current in the water. Because, the electrical current in water is transported by the ions present in them, and the conductivity is said to increase with the increase in the concentration of ions in them.

8.6.7.   Acidity

Acidity is the quantitative expression of water's capacity to neutralize a strong base to a designated pH and an indicator of how corrosive water is. Acidity can be caused by weak organic acids, such as acetic and tannic acids, and strong mineral acids including sulfuric and hydrochloric acids; however, the most common source of acidity in unpolluted water is carbon dioxide in the form of carbonic acid.

Acidity is classified by the pH value of a titration end point. Acidity caused by mineral acids exhibits a pH below 4.5. Salts of certain metals, particularly those with trivalent iron and aluminum, may hydrolyze in water and also contribute to acidity.

Acidity is commonly determined using methyl orange as a color indicator of the pH end point. Because methyl orange undergoes a color change from red to orange at a pH of 3.7, the results of the titration are termed Methyl Orange Acidity. Hach procedures for acidity use bromphenol blue indicator instead of methyl orange because the methyl orange color change is difficult to detect. The bromphenol blue indicator gives a sharp end point change from yellow to blue-violet.

Total acidity includes acidity caused by mineral acids, weak organic acids, and carbon dioxide (in the form of carbonic acid). Acidity determined by titrating to a phenolphthalein end point pH of 8.3 corresponds to the neutralization of carbonic acid to bicarbonate. Because carbon dioxide is the major cause of acidity in natural waters, in most cases the phenolphthalein acidity is equal to the total acidity. Acidity tests can be performed using a pH meter to detect the end points; however, methyl orange acidity and phenolphthalein acidity are the

8.6.8.   Alkalinity

Alkalinity is water's capacity to resist acidic changes in pH, essentially alkalinity is water's ability to neutralize acid. This ability is referred to as a buffering capacity. A water body with a high level of alkalinity (which is different than an alkaline water body) has higher levels of calcium carbonate, $CaCO_3$, which can decrease the water's acidity. Therefore, alkalinity measures how much acid can be added to a water body before a large pH change occurs.

One common method for measuring alkalinity is to use take a water sample and to add acid to it while checking the pH of the water as the acid is added. An initial pH reading of the water is taken and then small amounts of acid are added in increments, the water is stirred, and the pH is taken. This is done many times. In the beginning, the acid added will be neutralized by compounds in the water, such as bicarbonates. As more acid is added, the bicarbonates get "used up", as it is also being neutralized by the acid. Eventually all the acid-neutralizing compounds are used up. After this point, any acid added to the water will lower the pH in a linear fashion, and the scientist will be able to see this reflection point by viewing a line chart of the amount of acid added to the water and the resulting pH. The point at which the change in pH line becomes linear is used to determine the water's alkalinity.

8.7. Temperature

A temperature is a comparative objective measure of hot and cold. It is measured, typically by a thermometer, through the bulk behavior of a thermometric material, detection of heat radiation, or by particle velocity or kinetic energy. It may be calibrated in any of various temperature scales, Celsius, Fahrenheit, Kelvin, etc.

Temperature Conversion Instructions

The formulas used to convert between temperatures and as follows:

- Celsius to Fahrenheit: $°F = (°C * 9/5) + 32$ or, $°F = (°C * 1.8) + 32$
- Fahrenheit to Celsius: $°C = (°F - 32) * 5/9$ or, $°C = (°F - 32) / 1.8$
- Celsius to Kelvin: $K = °C + 273.15$
- Kelvin to Celsius: $°C = K = 273.15$
- Fahrenheit to Kelvin: $K = (°F + 459.67) * 5/9$
- Kelvin to Fahrenheit: $°F = K * 9/5 - 459.67$

9. Gravimetric Analysis

Gravimetric analysis is the process which describes a set of methods in analytical chemistry for the quantitative determination of an analyte based on the mass of a solid. E.g., the measurement of solids suspended in a water sample. A known volume of water is filtered and the collected solids are weighed.

A lot of measurements can be done by gravimetric analysis, and some of them are-

1) % Al_2O_3 in alum,
2) Ash content in coal,
3) Moisture content in coal,
4) Sulfated ash in corn flower,
5) Composition of white metal,
6) Composition of brass/bronze/gun metal,
7) Fe-, Al-content in cement,
8) Tin content in commercial tin,
9) Different cations such as-
   a. Al^{3+} and 8- hydroxyquinolate $Al(C_9H_6ON)_3$,
   b. Bi^{3+} as oxyiodide BiOl,
   c. NH4 as tetraphenylborate $NH4[B(C_6H_5)_4]$, etc.
10) Different anions such as-
   a. Cl^- as AgCL,
   b. F^- as PbCIF,
   c. SO_4^{2-} as $BaSO_4$, etc.

9.1. Chemical Factor or Gravimetric Factor

Chemical factor (also gravimetric factor) is defined as the stoichiometric ratio of molar mass of a species sought (element, ion, radical, compound, etc.) to that of the compound precipitated and weighed. The multiplication of the mass of the precipitate by gravimetric factor gives the mass of the species sought. So, it is very important in gravimetric analysis.

9.2. Steps Followed in the Gravimetric Analysis

- Preparation of a solution containing a known weight of the sample.
- Separation of the desired constituent.
- Weighing the isolated constituent.
- Computation of the amount of the particular constituent in the sample from the observed weight of the isolated substance.

9.3. Methods Involved in Gravimetric Analysis

The most important methods described in gravimetric analysis are-

a. **Precipitation**: The constituent being determined is precipitated from solution in a form which is so slightly soluble that no appreciable loss occurs when the precipitate is separated by filtration and weighed.

b. **Volatilization or evolution**: It depends essentially upon the removal of volatile constituents. This may be affected in several ways such as

       (i) Ignition in air or in a current of an indifferent gas,

(ii) Treatment with some chemical reagent whereby the desired constituent is rendered volatile,

(iii) Treatment with a chemical reagent whereby the desired constituent is rendered non-volatile.

c. **Electroanalytical**: The element to be determined is deposited electrolytical upon a suitable electrode. Electro-deposition is governed by Ohm's Law and Faraday's two Laws of Electrolysis.

d. **Extraction & chromatographic**: In liquid-liquid extraction, a solution (usually aqueous) is brought into contact with a second solvent (usually organic), essentially immiscible with the first, in order to bring about a transfer of one or more solutes into the second solvent. Chromatography is a separation process employed for the separation of mixtures of substances. GC and HPLC are used to make quantitative determinations.

9.4. The Procedure of Precipitation Methods

1. The sample is dissolved, if it is not already insoluble,
2. The solution is treated to adjust the pH. The sample may require treatment with different reagent to remove interferent,
3. The solution is heated gently to go the precipitate in colloidal form,
4. The precipitating reagent is added at a concentration that favors the formation of a good precipitate. This may require lowering the concentration,
5. The precipitate is allowed to digest at a higher temperature (usually on water bath),

6. The solution is filtered with a piece of ash less filter paper,
7. The precipitate- including the ash less filter pater on crucible – is heated. This achieves three purposes:
    i) Drying of precipitate,
    ii) Conversion of precipitate into a more chemically stable form,
    iii) Filter pater has burned away.
8. The precipitate is allowed to cool (perfectly in a desiccator) and then it is weighed as a pure compound.

9.5. Co-Precipitation

Co-precipitation is the phenomenon is which impurities, normally soluble in the mother liquor, and carried down along with the desired constituent. We cannot avoid co-precipitation; we can only minimize it by careful precipitation and through washing. Co-precipitation occurs due to

1. Adsorption of some unwanted particles at the surface of the precipitate,
2. The occlusion (entrapment withing the crustal) of foreign substances during the process of crystal growth from the primary particles.

9.6. Precipitate Completion Test

Precipitation completion test is performed by adding few drops of the precipitating reagent in the solution by the side of breaker without disturbing the settled precipitate: the upper part of solution being clear indicates the completion of precipitate. If some precipitates form, we need to add more precipitating reagent gently until it is seemed to be completed.

9.7. Digestion or Precipitate Ageing

Digestion (or precipitate ageing) means heating the precipitate along with the supernatant solution (or mother liquor) below its boiling point for about 12-24 hours. It results in cleaner and bigger particles. The physio-chemical process underlying digestion is called Ostwald ripening: an observed phenomenon in solid solutions or liquid sols which describes the change of and inhomogeneous structure over time, i.e., small crystals or sol particles dissolve, and redeposit onto larger crystals or particles.

9.8. Ignition

Ignition is the heating of precipitate (usually at 250-1200 $^\circ$C) to have a pure crystal of constant mass with the removal of water, volatile component and filter ash. After a precipitate has been filtered and washed, it must be ignited to constant composition before it can be weighed. Precipitates may contain-

1. Absorbed water on all solid surfaces,
2. Occluded water in cavities withing crystal,
3. Sorbed water in a large internal surface of crystal,
4. Essential water as in hydration and crystallization.

9.9. Advantages of Gravimetric Analysis:

1.   It is accurate and precise when using modern analytical balance.

2.   Possible sources of error are readily checked since filtrates can be tested for completeness of precipitation and precipitates may be examined for the presence of impurities.

3.   It is an absolute method; it involves direct measurement without any form of calibration being required.

4.   Determination can be carried out with relatively inexpensive apparatus; the most expensive items are a muffle furnace and sometimes platinum crucibles.

5.   Gravimetric analysis was used to determine the atomic masses of many elements to six figure accuracy.

6.   Gravimetry provides very little room for instrumental error and does not require a series of standards for calculation of an unknown.

9.10. **Disadvantage of Gravimetric method:**

1.   The chief disadvantage is that it requires meticulous time consuming.

2.   The chemist often prefers modern instrumental methods when they can be used.

3.   Gravimetric analysis usually only provides for the analysis of a single element, or a limited group of elements, at a time.

4.   Methods are often convoluted and a slight mis-step in a procedure can often mean disaster for the analysis (colloid formation in precipitation gravimetry, for example).

5.   Gravimetric analysis is based on the measurement of mass.

10. Titrimetric Analysis

Titration is a process of chemical analysis in which the quantity of some constituent of a sample is determined by adding to the measured sample an exactly known quantity of another substance with which the desired constituent reacts in a definite, known proportion. The process is usually carried out by gradually adding a standard solution (i.e., a solution of known concentration) of titrating reagent, or titrant, from a burette, essentially a long, graduated measuring tube with a stopcock and a delivery tube at its lower end. The addition is stopped when the equivalence point is reached.

Equivalence point: It is the point in titration at which the amount of titrant added is just enough to completely neutralize the analyte solution

End Point: The experimental point at which the completion of the reaction is marked by some signal is called the end point.

The difference between the end point and the equivalence point is the titration error, which is kept as small as possible by the proper choice of an end-point signal and a method for detecting it.

Indicator: It is the auxiliary reagent which detects the visual end point of a titration by some of its physical change, especially color.

There are different types of indicators

1. Neutralization Indicator
2. Adsorption Indicator
3. Redox Indicator
4. Metal ion Indicator
5. Zeta potential, etc.

Titrant: It is a solution of known concentration that is added (titrated) to another solution to determine the concentration of a second chemical species. The titrant may also be called the titrator, the reagent, or the standard solution.

Titrand: It is the unknown concentration of solution used during a titration. When a known concentration and volume of titrant is reacted with the analyte, it's possible to determine the analyte concentration.

10.1. Types of Titration

There are many types of titrations with different procedures and goals.

1. Acid–base titration
2. Redox titration
3. Gas phase titration
4. Complexometric titration
5. Zeta potential titration
6. Assay

Acid–base titration

An acid–base titration is a method of quantitative analysis for determining the concentration of an acid or base by exactly neutralizing it with a standard solution of base or acid having known concentration. A pH indicator is used to monitor the progress of the acid–base reaction. If the acid dissociation constant (pKa) of the acid or base dissociation constant (pKb) of base in the analyte solution is known, its solution concentration (molarity) can be determined. Alternately, the pKa can be determined if the analyte solution has a known solution concentration by constructing a titration curve.

Redox titration

A redox titration is a type of titration based on a redox reaction between the analyte and titrant. It may involve the use of a redox indicator and/or a potentiometer. A common example of a redox titration is treating a solution of iodine with a reducing agent to produce iodide using a starch indicator to help detect the endpoint. Iodine (I_2) can be reduced to iodide (I^-) by e.g. thiosulfate ($S_2O_3^{2-}$), and when all iodine is spent the blue color disappears. This is called an iodometric titration.

Gas phase titration

Gas phase titrations are titrations done in the gas phase, specifically as methods for determining reactive species by reaction with an excess of some other gas, acting as the titrant. In one common gas phase titration, gaseous ozone is titrated with nitrogen oxide according to the reaction

$$O_3 + NO \rightarrow O_2 + NO_2.$$

After the reaction is complete, the remaining titrant and product are quantified (e.g., by Fourier transform spectroscopy) (FT-IR); this is used to determine the amount of analyte in the original sample.

Complexometric titration

Complexometric titrations rely on the formation of a complex between the analyte and the titrant. In general, they require specialized complexometric indicators that form weak complexes with the analyte. The most common example is the use of starch indicator to increase the sensitivity of iodometric titration, the dark blue complex of starch with iodine and iodide being more visible than iodine alone. Other complexometric indicators are Eriochrome Black T for the titration of calcium and magnesium ions, and the chelating agent EDTA used to titrate metal ions in solution.

Zeta potential titration

Zeta potential titrations are titrations in which the completion is monitored by the zeta potential, rather than by an indicator, in order to characterize heterogeneous systems, such as colloids. One of the uses is to determine the iso-electric point when surface charge becomes zero, achieved by changing the pH or adding surfactant. Another use is to determine the optimum dose for flocculation or stabilization

Assay

An assay is a type of biological titration used to determine the concentration of a virus or bacterium. Serial dilutions are performed on a sample in a fixed ratio (such as 1:1, 1:2, 1:4, 1:8, etc.) until the last dilution does not give a positive test for the presence of the virus. The positive or negative value may be determined by inspecting the infected cells visually under a microscope or by an immunoenzymetric method such as enzyme-linked immunosorbent assay (ELISA).

10.2. Primary Standard

Primary Standard is a reagent of sufficient purity from which a standard solution can be prepared by direct weighing of a quantity of it.

The solution produced by a primary standard is called primary standard solution.

Characteristics of a primary standard include

1. High purity
2. Stability
3. Low reactivity
4. Low hygroscopicity and efflorescence
5. High solubility
6. High molar mass
7. Non toxicity
8. Ready to cheap availability
9. Eco-friendliness

The substances commonly employed as primary standard are listed below

I. Acid Base reaction : Na_2CO_3, Potassium Hydrogen phthalate
II. Complexometric reaction: Ag, $AgNO_3$, NaCl
III. Precipitation reaction: Ag, $AgNO_3$, NaCl
IV. Redox reaction: $K_2Cr_2O_7$, KIO_3, $KBrO_3$

10.3. Secondary Standard

Secondary standard is a reagent which may be used for standardization and whose content of active substance has been found by comparison against primary standard.

The solution in which the concentration of dissolve solute has not been determined from the weight of the compound dissolved but by reaction of a volume of the solution against a measured volume of a primary standard solution is called the secondary standard solution.

11. Chromatography

Chromatography is a laboratory_technique for the separation of a mixture. The mixture is dissolved in a fluid called the mobile phase, which carries it through a structure holding another material called the stationary phase. The various constituents of the mixture travel at different speeds, causing them to separate. The separation is based on differential partitioning between the mobile and stationary phases.

11.1. Chromatographic Terms

Stationary phase: This phase is always composed of a "solid" phase or "a layer of a liquid adsorbed on the surface solid support".

Mobile phase: This phase is always composed of "liquid" or a "gaseous component."

Chromatograph: Equipment that enables a sophisticated separation EX. Gas chromatography or Liquid chromatography

Eluent: Fluid entering column/ solvent that carries the analyte.

Eluate: Mobile phase leaving the column.

Retention time: It is the characteristic time it takes for a particular analyte to pass through the system (from the column inlet to the detector) under set conditions.

11.2. Principles of Chromatography

Chromatography is a separation method where the analyte is combined within a liquid or gaseous mobile phase. which is pumped through a stationary phase. Usually one phase is hydrophilic and the other lipophilic. The components of the analyte interact differently with these two phases. Depending of their polarity and separation of fractions of mixture based on their relative affinity towards the two phases during their travel. The fraction with greater affinity to stationary phase travels slower and shorter while that with less affinity travels faster and longer. The separation is based on Differential partitioning between the mobile and stationary phases.

They spend more or less time interacting with the stationary phase and are thus retarded to a greater or lesser extend. This leads to the separation of the different components present in the sample. Each sample component elutes from the stationary phase at a specific time, its retention time. As the components pass through the detector their signal is recorded and plotted in the form of a chromatogram.

11.3. Type of Chromatography

Column chromatography: In this type, the stationary phase is packed into a glass or metal columns (wide tubes or cylinders). The mixture to be separated is layered on the top of the column in the form of a solution at particular concentration. After equilibration the components are eluted out of the column one by one using specific mobile phases (Fig.10.2). The solvent used to elute the separated components is known as eluant.

Thin layer chromatography: In this type, the stationary phase is thinly coated on to a glass, plastic or foil plates. The mixture to be separated is applied on the stationary phase at one end and kept vertical in the petridish containing the mobile phase. When the mobile phase reaches the other end of the plate the plate is removed from the petridish and the compounds separated are identified by using specific staining reagents

Paper chromatography: In this type, the stationary **column chromatography** phase is supported by the cellulose fibres of a paper sheet. The mobile phase flows through the stationary phase and effects separation.

 Column Chromatography:

All the major types of chromatography are routinely carried out using column type (Fig. 10.3). The different types of column chromatography are

1) adsorption chromatography
2) partition chromatography
3) ion-exchange chromatography
4) exclusion chromatography
5) affinity chromatography

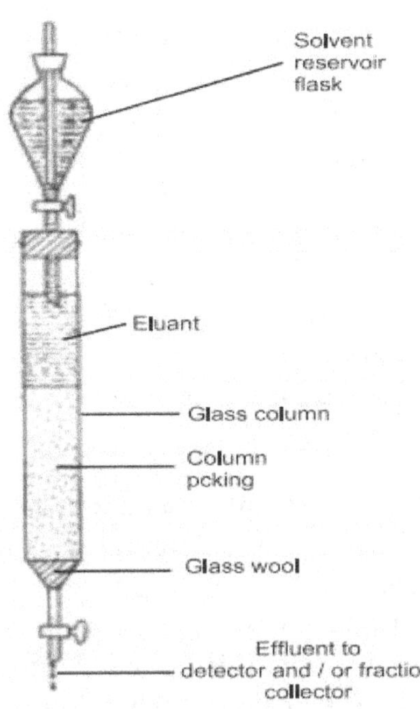

Adsorption chromatography

An adsorbent may be described as a solid which has the property of adsorbing molecules at its surface, particularly when it is porous and finely divided. Adsorption can be specific so that one solute may be adsorbed selectively from a mixture. Separation of components by the method depends upon differences both in their degree of adsorption by the adsorbent and solubility in the solvent used for separation. Adsorption chromatography can be carried out in both the column and thin layer modes.

Partition chromatography

This technique is based on the partitioning of compounds between a liquid stationary phase and a liquid mobile phase. The liquid stationary phase can be held on any solid support like paper. This technique is otherwise known as liquid- liquid chromatography.

Gas liquid chromatography

This technique is based upon the partitioning of compounds between a liquid stationary phase and a gas mobile phase . It is a widely used method for the qualitative and quantitative analysis of a large number of compounds (eg. fatty acids) because it has high sensitivity, reproducibility and speed of resolution. A stationary phase of liquid material such as a silicone grease is supported on an inert granular solid. This material is packed into a narrow-coiled glass or steel column 1 to 3 meter long and 2 to 4mm internal diameter. Through this column an inert carrier gas (the mobile phase) such as nitrogen, helium or argon is passed. The column is maintained in an oven at an elevated temperature which volatilizes the compounds to be separated.

The basis for the separation is the difference in the partition coefficients of the volatilized compounds between the liquid and gas phases as the compounds are carried through the column by the carrier gas. As the compounds flow, they leave the column and pass through a detector which is connected to a recorder and record a peak. The area of the peak corresponds to the concentration of the compound separated.

Ion exchange chromatography

The principle of this form of chromatography is the attraction between oppositely charged particles. Many biological materials, such as amino acids and proteins, have ionizable groups and the fact that may carry a net positive or negative charge can be utilized in separating mixtures of such compounds. The net charge carried by such compounds depend on their pKa and on the pH of the solution.

Ion exchange separations are mainly carried out in columns packed with an ion exchanger, which contain the core matrix molecule with exchangeable ionic groups on its surface. There are two types of ion exchangers, namely cation and anion exchangers. Cation exchangers posses negatively charged groups and they will attract positively charged molecules. Anion exchangers have positively charged groups which will attract negatively charged molecules. The actual ion exchange mechanism composed of four steps;

- selective adsorption of the molecules to be separated by the ion exchange resins. B release of the exchangeable group from the matrix.

- Elution of the absorbed molecule by specific eluants.

- Regeneration of the matrix by recharging with the original exchangeable groups.

Cation exchanger

$$RSO_3\text{----------}Na^+ \; + (X^+, X, Y) \xrightarrow{\text{adsorbtion}} RSO_3\text{-----}X^+ + Na^+$$
(exchanger counter mixture of compounds)

(elution)

$$RSO_3\text{-----}X^+ + H^+ \Longrightarrow RSO_3\text{-------}H^+ + X^+ \text{(separated ion)}$$

$$RSO_3\text{-------}H^+ + NaCl \Longrightarrow RSO_3\text{-------}Na^+ + HCl$$
(recharging)

Anion exchanger

$$R\,NH_3 \text{----------} OH^- + (X^-, X, Y) \Longrightarrow RNH_3\text{-----}X^- + OH^-$$
(mixture of compounds)

(elution)

$$RNH_3\text{-----}X^- + Cl^- \Longrightarrow RNH_3\text{-----}Cl^- + X^- \text{ (separated ion)}$$

$$OH\, RNH_3\text{-----}Cl^- + OH^- \Longrightarrow RNH_3\text{-----}OH^- + Cl^-$$
(recharging)

Some of the ion exchange materials used in this technique are Amberlite IRC 50, Bio- Rex, Dowex 50, Sephadex etc.

Molecular exclusion chromatography

This chromatography is otherwise known as gel permeation chromatography.

This technique is based on the separation of molecules on the basis of their molecular size and shape and the molecular sieve properties of a variety of porous materials which serve as the solid stationary phase.

A column of gel particles or porous glass granules is in equilibrium with a suitable solvent for the molecules to be separated. Large molecules which are completely excluded from the pores will pass through the interstitial spaces and smaller molecules will be distributed between the solvent inside and outside the molecular sieve and will then pass through the column at a lower rate. So the larger particles will come out of the column first followed by smaller particles.

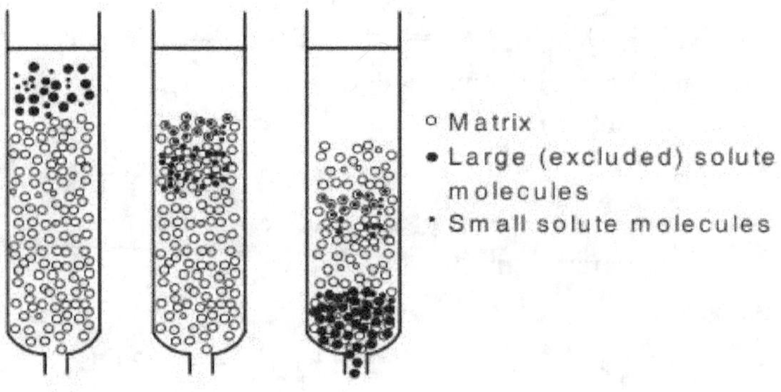

Fig. 10.4 Diagrammatic representation of separation by exclusive chromatography

The gel materials generally used for this technique are cross-linked dextrans, agarose, polyacrylamide, poly styrene etc.

Affinity chromatography:

This technique is based on the specific biological interaction of the compounds to be separated with the special molecules attached on the stationary phase called as ligands. This technique requires that the material to be isolated is capable of reversibly binding to a specific ligand which is attached to an insoluble matrix (stationary phase).

$$M \quad + \quad L \quad \rightleftharpoons \quad ML$$

macro-molecule   ligand (attached to matrix)   Complex

Under suitable experimental conditions when a complex mixture containing the specific compound to be purified is added to the insolubilized ligand generally contained in a chromatography column, only that compound will bind to the ligand. All the other compounds can be washed away and the compound subsequently recovered by displacement from the ligand. The purification of an enzyme by this technique is shown diagrammatically below.

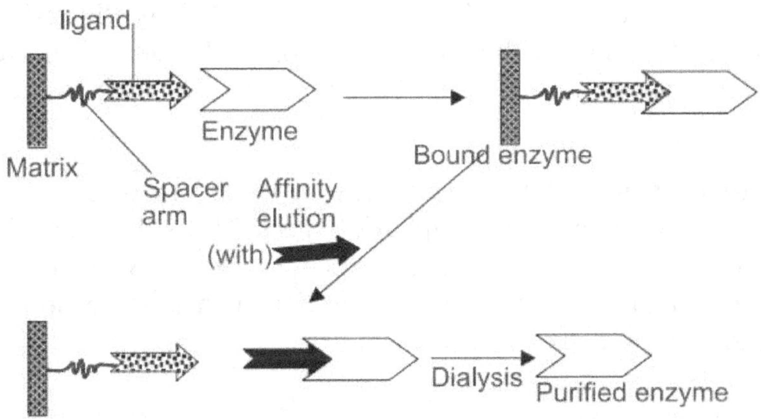

In practice, particles which are uniform, spherical and rigid are used as matrix materials such as polystyrene, cellulose, porous glass and silica etc.

11.3.2.   Thin Layer Chromatography

Principle: Partition, adsorption, exclusion chromatography can be carried out in a thin layer mode. In this technique the stationary phase is made in the form of a slurry and applied as a thin coating on the surface of a glass plate. After activating the plate, the sample to be separated is applied at one end of the plate . The plate is kept vertically in a chamber specially designed for this purpose (TLC chamber) and

99

allowed the sample and the mobile phase to raise through the stationary phase by capillary action. The whole procedure consists of.

a. Thin layer preparation =: A slurry of the stationary phase, generally applied to a glass, plastic or foil plate as a uniform thin layer by means of a plate spreader starting from one end of the plate and moving progressively to the other. Calcium phosphate is incorporated into the slurry in order to facilitate the adhesion of the adsorbent to the plate. The plate is heated in an oven at 1000 C to activate the adsorbent.

b. Sample application: The sample is applied to the plate by means of a micropipette or syringe as spot or as a band on the stationary phase.

c. Plate development: Separation takes place in a glass tank which contains mobile phase to a depth of about 1.5 cm. This is allowed to stand for at least an hour with a lid over the top of the tank to ensure that the atmosphere within the tank becomes saturated with solvent vapour.

d. Component detection: The components separated are detected by (i) spraying the plate with 50% sulphuric acid or 25% sulphuric acid in ethanol and heating; (ii) examining the plate under ultraviolet light; (iii) spraying of plates with specific colour reagents, for example ninhydrin for amino acids.

11.3.3.   Paper Chromatography

The cellulose fibers of chromatography paper act as the supporting matrix for the stationary phase. The stationary phase may be water or a non-polar material such as liquid paraffin. The components get separated between the liquid stationary phase and the liquid mobile phase. The procedure consists of

a. Paper development: There are two techniques which may be employed for the development of paper, ascending and descending methods. In both cases, the solvent is placed in the base of a sealed tank or glass jar to allow the chamber to become saturated with the solvent paper. The sample spots should be in a position just above the surface of the solvent so that as the solvent moves vertically up the paper by capillary action, separation of the sample is achieved.

b. Component detection: The separated components can be detected by (i) examining the paper under ultraviolet light; (ii) spraying of papers with specific color reagents, for example ninhydrin for amino acids and sulphuric acid for simple sugars.

The identification of a given compound may be made on the basis of its R_f value (retardation factor) which is the distance moved by the component during development divided by the distance moved by the solvent from the point of origin

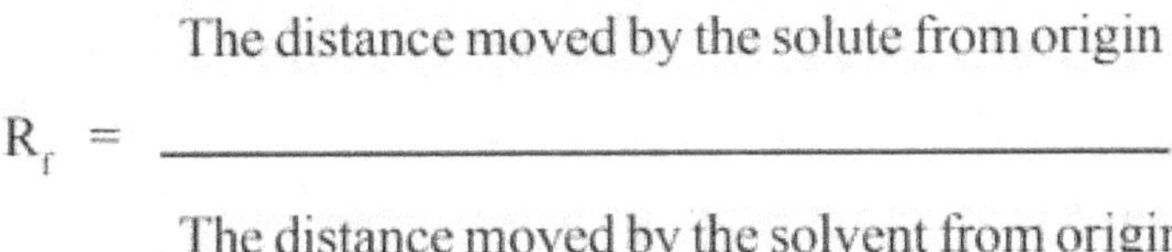

$$R_f = \frac{\text{The distance moved by the solute from origin}}{\text{The distance moved by the solvent from origin}}$$

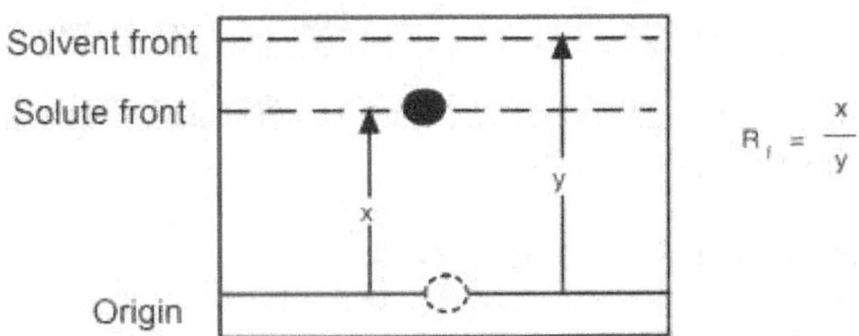

The value of R_f is constant for a particular compound under standard conditions and closely reflects the distribution co-efficient for that compound.

11.4. The Advantages of Chromatography

- Precise separation, analyses, and purification is possible using chromatography.
- It requires very low sample volumes.

- It works on a wide range of samples including drugs, food particles, plastics, pesticides, air and water samples, and tissue extracts.
- Mixture components separated by chromatography can be collected individually.
- It can be used to separate highly complex mixtures.

11.5. Applications of Chromatography

Pharmaceutical sector

- To identify and analyze samples for the presence of trace elements or chemicals.
- Separation of compounds based on their molecular weight and element composition.
- Detects the unknown compounds and purity of mixture.
- In drug development.

Chemical industry

- In testing water samples and also checks air quality.
- HPLC and GC are very much used for detecting various contaminants such as polychlorinated biphenyl (PCBs) in pesticides and oils.

In various life sciences applications

Food Industry

- In food spoilage and additive detection
- Determining the nutritional quality of food

Forensic Science

- In forensic pathology and crime scene testing like analyzing blood and hair samples of crime place.

Molecular Biology Studies

- Various hyphenated techniques in chromatography such as EC-LC-MS are applied in the study of metabolomics and proteomics along with nucleic acid research.

- HPLC is used in Protein Separation like Insulin Purification, Plasma Fractionation, and Enzyme Purification and also in various departments like Fuel Industry, biotechnology, and biochemical processes.

12. Spectroscopy

Spectroscopy is the investigation and measurement of spectra produced by matter interacting with or emitting electromagnetic radiation. Originally, spectroscopy was defined as the study of the interaction between radiation and matter as a function of wavelength. Now, spectroscopy is defined as any measurement of a quantity as a function of wavelength or frequency. During a spectroscopy experiment, electromagnetic radiation of a specified wavelength range passes from a source through a sample containing compounds of interest, resulting in absorption or emission. During absorption, the sample absorbs energy from the light source. During emission, the sample emits light of a different wavelength than the source's wavelength

12.1. Spectrophotometer

The spectrophotometer is an instrument which measures an amount of light that a sample absorbs. The spectrophotometer works by passing a light beam through a sample to measure the light intensity of a sample. These instruments are used in the process of measuring color and used for monitoring color accuracy throughout production. They are primarily used by researchers and manufacturers everywhere. The major Spectrophotometer applications are limitless as they are used in practically every industrial and commercial field. However, it finds its major applications in liquids, plastics, paper, metals and fabrics. This helps in ensuring that the color chosen remains consistent from its original conception to the final, finished product.

Electromagnetic radiation can be divided into seven distinct regions.

Region	Frequency	Wavelength
Radio	$< 3 \times 10^9$ Hz	> 10 cm
Microwave	$3 \times 10^9 - 3 \times 10^{11}$ Hz	$10 - 0.1$ cm
Infrared	$3 \times 10^{11} - 4 \times 10^{14}$ Hz	$1000 - 0.7$ μm
Visible	$4 \times 10^{14} - 7.5 \times 10^{14}$ Hz	$700 - 400$ nm
Ultraviolet	$7.5 \times 10^{14} - 3 \times 10^{16}$ Hz	$400 - 10$ nm
X-ray	$3 \times 10^{16} - 3 \times 10^{19}$ Hz	$10 - 0.01$ nm
γ-ray	$> 3 \times 10^{19}$ Hz	< 0.01 nm

12.2.   Types of Spectrophotometer

Spectrophotometer is of 2 types

- Single beam spectrophotometer

- Double beam spectrophotometer

Single beam spectrophotometer operates between 325 nm to 1000 nm wavelength using the single beam of light. The light travels in one direction and the test solution and blank are read in the same.

Double beam spectrophotometer operates between 185 nm to 1000 nm wavelength. It has two photocells. This instrument splits the light from the Monochromator into two beams. One beam is used for reference and the other for sample reading. It eliminates the error which occurs due to fluctuations in the light output and the sensitivity of the detector.

12.2.1.   Principle of Spectrophotometer

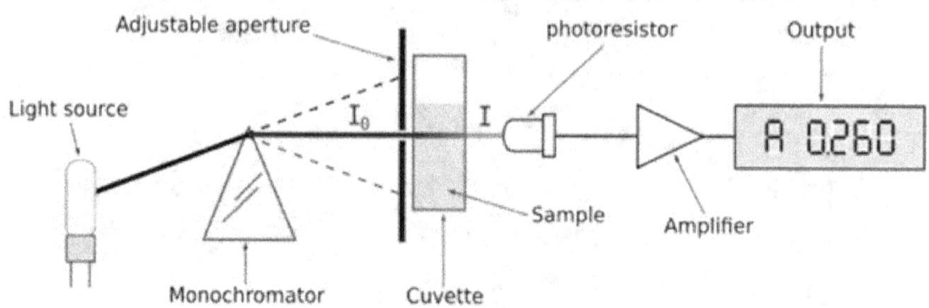

A spectrophotometer is made up of two instruments: a spectrometer and a photometer. The spectrometer is to produce light of any wavelength, while the photometer is to measure the intensity of light. The spectrophotometer is designed in a way that the liquid or a sample is placed between spectrometer and photometer. The photometer measures the amount of light that passes through the sample and delivers a voltage signal to the display. If the absorbing of light change, the voltage signal also changes. Spectrophotometers come in a variety of shapes and sizes and have multipurpose uses to them. The different types of spectrophotometers available are all different from one another, based on their application and desired functionality. Another closely related concept is spectroscopy that simply measures the absorption of light from its source and the intensity of light as well.

The intensity of light is symbolized as I_0 measure the number of photons per second. When the light is passed through the blank solution, it does not absorb light and is symbolized as (I). Other important factors are Absorbance (A) and Transmittance (T).

$$T = I_t/I_o$$

$$A = -\log_{10} T$$

Here, we need to measure the intensity of light that passes a blank solution, and later measures the intensity of light passing a sample.

Calculate the transmittance and the absorbance. For the measurement of absorbance, we can use an isosbestic point where the absorbance and wavelength of two or more species are the same.

A number of protons transmit and absorb totally depended on the length of the cuvette and the concentration of the sample.

The transmittance and absorption relation is:

$$\text{Absorbance (A)} = -\log(T) = -\log(T) = -\log(I_t/I_0)$$

The transmittance of an unknown sample can be calculated using the formula given below.

Transmittance $T = I_t/I_o$

Here,

I_t = Light intensity after passing via cuvette

I_0 = Light intensity before passing via cuvette

Further, there are several varieties of spectrophotometer devices such as UV Spectrometry, atomic emission spectrophotometry and atomic absorption spectrophotometry and much more. It can also be classified into two types based on the range of light source wavelengths like IR spectrophotometer and UV-visible spectrophotometer. Some of the major real life applications of spectrophotometry in various fields are laundry soap, carpeting and production of small parts such as toys or intricate machinery. The major types of spectrophotometers are categorized into 2, these are mainly portable spectrophotometers and bench spectrophotometers, they both are unique and have their own uses.

12.3. Beer Lambert's Law

Beer's Law

$\Rightarrow$ This law states that the amount of light absorbed is directly proportional to the concentration of the solute in the solution.

$$\text{Log}_{10}\ I_0/I_1 = a_s c$$

where,

I_O = Intensity of primary light

I_1 = Intensity of passing light

a_s = Absorbency index

c = Concentration of Solution

Lambert's Law

$\Rightarrow$ The Lambert's law states that the amount of light absorbed is directly proportional to the length and thickness of the solution under analysis.

$$A = \log_{10}\ I_0/I_1 = a_s b$$

Where,

A = Absorbance of test

a_s = Absorbance of standard

b = length / thickness of the solution

The mathematical representation of the combined form of Beer-Lambert's law is as follows:

$$\text{Log}_{10}\ I_0\ /\ I_1 = a_s bc$$

If b is kept constant by applying Cuvette or standard cell then,

$$\text{Log}_{10}\ I_0/I_1 = a_s c$$

The absorbency index as is defined as= A/cl

Where,

c = concentration of the absorbing material (in gm/liter).

l = distance traveled by the light in solution (in cm).

In simplified form,

The working principle of the Spectrophotometer is based on Beer-Lambert's law which states that the amount of light absorbed by a color solution is directly proportional to the concentration of the solution and the length of a light path through the solution.

$A \propto cl$

Where,

A = Absorbance / Optical density of solution

c = Concentration of solution

l = Path length

or, $A = \epsilon cl$

ϵ = Absorption coefficient

Limitations of the Beer–Lambert law

The linearity of the Beer-Lambert law is limited by chemical and instrumental factors. Causes of nonlinearity include:

- Deviations in absorptivity coefficients at high concentrations (>0.01M) due to electrostatic interactions between molecules in close proximity
- Scattering of light due to particulates in the sample
- Fluoresecence or phosphorescence of the sample
- Changes in refractive index at high analyte concentration
- Shifts in chemical equilibria as a function of concentration

- Non-monochromatic radiation, deviations can be minimized by using a relatively flat part of the absorption spectrum such as the maximum of an absorption band

12.4. Types of Spectroscopy

There are mainly two types of spectroscopy

1) Atomic Spectroscopy
2) Molecular Spectroscopy

12.4.1. Atomic Spectroscopy

Atomic spectroscopy was the first application of spectroscopy developed, and it can be split into atomic absorption, emission and fluorescence spectroscopy. Atoms of different elements have distinct spectra so atomic spectroscopy can quantify and identify a sample's composition. The main types of atomic spectroscopy include atomic absorption spectroscopy (AAS), atomic emission spectroscopy (AES) and atomic fluorescence spectroscopy (AFS).

Atomic Absorption Spectroscopy (AAS)

In AAS atoms absorb ultraviolet or visible light to transition to higher levels of energy. AAS quantifies the amount of absorption of ground state atoms in the gaseous state. AAS is commonly used in the detection of metals.

Atomic Emission Spectroscopy (AES)

In AES, atoms are excited from the heat of a flame, plasma, arc or spark to emit light. AES used the intensity of light emitted to determine the quantity of an element in a sample. Techniques that use AES include flame emission spectroscopy, inductively coupled plasma atomic emission spectroscopy, and spark or arc atomic emission spectroscopy.

Atomic Fluorescence Spectroscopy (AFS).

In AFS, it is a beam of light that excites the analytes, causing them to emit light. The fluorescence from a sample is then analyzed using a fluorometer, and it is commonly used to analyze organic compounds.

12.4.2.   Molecular Spectrometer

Molecular spectroscopy relates to the interactions that occur between molecules and electromagnetic radiation. Electromagnetic radiation is a form of radiation in which the electric and magnetic fields simultaneously vary. One well known example of electromagnetic radiation is visible light. Electromagnetic radiation can be characterized by its energy, intensity, frequency and wavelength.

Different types of molecular spectroscopy are given below

Ultraviolet and Visible Spectroscopy

Ultraviolet (UV) and visible (Vis) spectroscopy analyses compounds using the electromagnetic radiation spectrum from 10 nm to 700 nm. Many atoms are able to emit or absorb visible light, and it is this absorption or reflectance that gives the apparent color of the chemicals being analyzed.

The absorption of visible and UV radiation is associated with excitation of electrons from a low energy ground state into a high energy excited state, and the energy can be absorbed by both non-bonding n-electrons and π-electrons within a molecular orbital.

Wavelengths of light all have a particular energy associated with them, and it is only light with the right amount of energy that causes transitions from one level to another for absorption. For larger gaps between energy levels, more energy is required for promotion to the higher energy level, so there will be higher frequency and shorter wavelength absorbed.

UV and visible spectroscopy can be used to measure the concentration of samples using the principles of the Beer-Lambert Law, which states that absorbance is proportional to the concentration of the substance in solution and the path length. As well as for measuring the concentration of a sample, UV and visible spectroscopy can be used to identify the presence of the free electrons and double bonds within a molecule. In addition to being an analytical technique that can be used alone, a UV/Vis spectrometer can be used as a detector for high-performance liquid chromatography.

Infrared Spectroscopy

Infrared (IR) analyses compounds using the infrared spectrum, which can be split into near IR, mid-IR and far IR. Near IR has the greatest energy and can penetrate a sample much deeper than mid or far IR, but due to this, it is also the least sensitive. Infrared spectroscopy is not as sensitive as UV/Vis spectroscopy due to the energies involved in the vibration of atoms being smaller than the energies of the transitions.

IR uses the principle that molecules vibrate, with bonds stretching and bending, when they absorb infrared radiation. IR spectroscopy works by passing a beam of IR light through a sample, and for an IR detectable transition, the molecules of the sample must undergo dipole moment change during vibration. When the frequency of the IR is the same as the vibrational frequency of the bonds, absorption occurs and a spectrum can be recorded.

Different functional groups absorb heat at different frequencies depending on their structure, and thus a vibrational spectrum can be used to determine the functional groups present in a sample. When interpreting the data obtained by an IR, results can be compared to a frequency table to find out which functional groups are present to help determine the structure.

Raman Spectroscopy

Raman spectroscopy is similar to IR in that it is a vibrational spectroscopy technique, but it uses inelastic scattering. The spectrum of Raman spectroscopy shows a scattered Rayleigh line and the Stoke and anti-Stoke lines, which is different from the irregular absorbance lines of IR.

Raman spectroscopy works by the detection of inelastic scattering, also known as Raman scattering, of monochromatic light from a laser in the visible, near-infrared or ultraviolet range. For a transition to be Raman active, there must be a change in the polarizability of the molecule during the vibration and the electron cloud must experience a positional change.

The technique provides a molecular fingerprint of the chemical composition and structures of samples, but Raman scattering gives inherently weak signals. Techniques such as Surface Enhanced Raman Spectroscopy (SERS) have been developed to enhance sensitivity when using Raman spectroscopy.

Nuclear Magnetic Resonance

Nuclear magnetic resonance (NMR) uses resonance spectroscopy and nuclear spin states for spectroscopic analysis. All nuclei have a nuclear spin, and the spin behavior of the nucleus of every atom depends on its intramolecular environment and the external applied field.

When nuclei of a particular element are in different chemical environments within the same molecule, there will be varied magnetic field strengths experienced due to shielding and de-shielding of electrons close by, causing different resonant frequencies and defines the chemical shift values.

Spin-spin coupling takes into account that the spin states of one nucleus affect the magnetic field that is experienced by neighboring nuclei, via intervening bonds. Spin-spin coupling causes absorption peaks of each group of nuclei to be split into a number of components.

There are multiple types of NMR analyses, which are hydrogen NMR, carbon 13 NMR, DEPT 90 and DEPT 135 NMR. The NMR spectrum of a compound shows the resonance signals that are emitted by the atomic nuclei present in a sample, and these can be used to identify the structure of a compound.

12.5. Instrumentation of Spectrophotometer

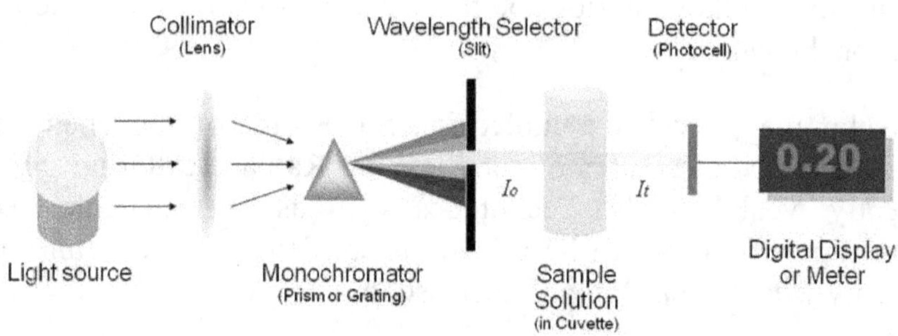

The essential components of spectrophotometer instrumentation include:

A table and cheap radiant energy source

Materials that can be excited to high energy states by a high voltage electric discharge (or) by electrical heating serve as excellent radiant energy sources.

Monochromator

A monochromator, to break the polychromatic radiation into component wavelength (or) bands of wavelengths. It resolves polychromatic radiation into its individual wavelengths and isolates these wavelengths into very narrow bands.

- Prisms:
  A prism disperses polychromatic light from the source into its constituent wavelengths by virtue of its ability to reflect different wavelengths to a different extent
  Two types of Prisms are usually employed in commercial instruments. Namely, 600 cornu quartz prism and 300 Littrow Prism.

- Grating:
  Gratings are often used in the monochromators of spectrophotometers operating ultraviolet, visible and infrared regions.

Transport vessels (cuvettes)

It is mainly used to hold the sample. Samples to be studied in the ultraviolet (or) visible region are usually glasses (or) solutions and are put in cells known as "CUVETTES". Cuvettes meant for the visible region are made up of either ordinary glass (or) sometimes Quartz.

A Photosensitive detector and an associated readout system

Most detectors depend on the photoelectric effect. The current is then proportional to the light intensity and therefore a measure of it.

Radiation detectors generate electronic signals which are proportional to the transmitter light. These signals need to be translated into a form that is easy to interpret. This is accomplished by using amplifiers, Ammeters, Potentiometers and Potentiometric recorders.

12.6. Applications of Spectrophotometer

Some of the major applications of spectrophotometers include the following:

- Detection of concentration of substances
- Detection of impurities
- Structure elucidation of organic compounds
- Monitoring dissolved oxygen content in freshwater and marine ecosystems
- Characterization of proteins
- Detection of functional groups
- Respiratory gas analysis in hospitals
- Molecular weight determination of compounds
- The visible and UV spectrophotometer may be used to identify classes of compounds in both the pure state and in biological preparations.

13. Polymer

A polymer is a large molecule or a macromolecule which essentially is a combination of many subunits. The term polymer in Greek means 'many parts. Polymers can be found all around us. From the strand of our DNA which is a naturally occurring biopolymer to polypropylene which is used throughout the world as plastic.

Polymers may be naturally found in plants and animals (**natural polymers**) or may be man-made (**synthetic polymers**). Different polymers have a number of unique physical and chemical properties due to which they find usage in everyday life.

13.1. Classification of Polymers

Polymers cannot be classified under one category because of their complex structures, different behaviors, and vast applications. We can, therefore, classify polymers based on the following considerations.

13.1.1. Classification Based on the Source of Availability

There are three types of classification under this category

1. Natural polymer
2. Synthetic polymer
3. Semi-synthetic Polymers.

Natural Polymers:

They occur naturally and are found in plants and animals. For example, proteins, starch, cellulose, and rubber. To add up, we also have biodegradable polymers which are called biopolymers.

Semi-synthetic Polymers:

They are derived from naturally occurring polymers and undergo further chemical modification. For example, cellulose nitrate, cellulose acetate.

Synthetic Polymers:

These are man-made polymers. Plastic is the most common and widely used synthetic polymer. It is used in industries and various dairy products. For example, nylon-6, 6, polyether's etc.

13.1.2. Classification Based on the Structure of the Monomer Chain

This category has the following classifications:

Linear Polymers

The structure of polymers containing long and straight chains fall into this category. PVC, i.e. poly-vinyl chloride is largely used for making pipes and electric cables is an example of a linear polymer.

Branched-chain Polymers

When linear chains of a polymer form branch, then, such polymers are categorized as branched chain polymers. For example, Low-density polythene.

Cross-linked Polymers

They are composed of bifunctional and trifunctional monomers. They have a stronger covalent bond in comparison to other linear polymers. Bakelite and melamine are examples in this category.

13.1.3. Classification Based on Polymerization

I.   Addition Polymerization: Example, poly ethane, Teflon, Polyvinyl chloride (PVC)
II. Condensation Polymerization: Example, Nylon -6, 6, perylene, polyesters.

13.1.4. Classification Based on Monomers

I. **Homomer**: In this type, a single type of monomer unit is present. For example, Polyethene

Heteropolymer or co-polymer: It consists of different type of monomer units. For example, nylon -6, 6

13.1.5. Classification Based on Molecular Forces

Elastomers: These are rubber-like solids weak interaction forces are present. For example, Rubber.

Fibers: Strong, tough, high tensile strength and strong forces of interaction are present. For example, nylon -6, 6.

Thermoplastics: These have intermediate forces of attraction. For example, polyvinyl chloride.

Thermosetting polymers: These polymers greatly improve the material's mechanical properties. It provides enhanced chemical and heat resistance. For example, phenolics, epoxies, and silicones.

13.2. Structure of Polymers

Most of the polymers around us are made up of a hydrocarbon backbone. A Hydrocarbon backbone being a long chain of linked carbon and hydrogen atoms, possible due to the tetravalent nature of carbon.

A few examples of a hydrocarbon backbone polymer are polypropylene, polybutylene, polystyrene. Also, there are polymers which instead of carbon have other elements in its backbone. For example, Nylon, which contains nitrogen atoms in the repeated unit backbone.

13.3. **Properties of Polymers**

13.3.1. Physical Properties

- As chain length and cross-linking increases the tensile strength of the polymer increases.
- Polymers do not melt; they change state from crystalline to semi-crystalline.

13.3.2. Chemical Properties

- Compared to conventional molecules with different side molecules, the polymer is enabled with hydrogen bonding and ionic bonding resulting in better cross-linking strength.
- Dipole-dipole bonding side chains enable the polymer for high flexibility.
- Polymers with Van der Waals forces linking chains are known to be weak, but give the polymer a low melting point.

13.3.3. Optical Properties

- Due to their ability to change their refractive index with temperature as in the case of PMMA and HEMA: MMA, they are used in lasers for applications in spectroscopy and analytical applications.

13.4. **Some Polymers and their Monomers**

- Polypropene, also known as polypropylene, is made up of monomer propene.
- Polystyrene is an aromatic polymer, naturally transparent, made up of monomer styrene.
- Polyvinyl chloride (PVC) is a plastic polymer made of monomer vinyl chloride.
- The urea-formaldehyde resin is a non-transparent plastic obtained by heating formaldehyde and urea.
- Glyptal is made up of monomers ethylene glycol and phthalic acid.
- Bakelite or polyoxybenzylmethylenglycolanhydride is a plastic which is made up of monomers phenol and aldehyde.

13.5. Types of Polymerization Reactions

Addition Polymerization

This is also called as chain growth polymerization. In this, small monomer units joined to form a giant polymer. In each step length of chain increases. For example, Polymerization of ethane in the presence of Peroxides

Condensation Polymerization

In this type small molecules like H_2O, CO, NH_3 are eliminated during polymerization (step growth polymerization). Generally, organic compounds containing bifunctional groups such as idols, -dials, diamines, dicarboxylic acids undergo this type of polymerization reaction. For example, Preparation of nylon -6, 6.

13.6. Uses of Polymers

Here we will list some of the important uses of polymers in our everyday life.

- Polypropene finds usage in a broad range of industries such as textiles, packaging, stationery, plastics, aircraft, construction, rope, toys, etc.
- Polystyrene is one of the most common plastic, actively used in the packaging industry. Bottles, toys, containers, trays, disposable glasses and plates, tv cabinets and lids are some of the daily-used products made up of polystyrene. It is also used as an insulator.
- The most important use of polyvinyl chloride is the manufacture of sewage pipes. It is also used as an insulator in the electric cables.
- Polyvinyl chloride is used in clothing and furniture and has recently become popular for the construction of doors and windows as well. It is also used in vinyl flooring.
- Urea-formaldehyde resins are used for making adhesives, moulds, laminated sheets, unbreakable containers, etc.

- Glyptal is used for making paints, coatings, and lacquers.
- Bakelite is used for making electrical switches, kitchen products, toys, jewellery, firearms, insulators, computer discs, etc.

13.7. Polymers vs Plastics

Although the words 'polymer' and 'plastic' are typically used interchangeably, plastics are literally only 1 reasonably chemical compound. They're polymers that have malleability. In different words, they'll be molded—using heat, as an example.

Many plastics are synthesized from hydrocarbon-containing oil or rock oil (though not all plastics are: bioplastics, as an example, is made up of plants or perhaps bacteria). The method by that oil is was plastic usually goes one thing like this. First, a refinery cracks the oil into little hydrocarbons (the monomers). An organic compound plant receives the monomers and, mistreatment the processes that we'll describe during a moment, these are reacted to become polymers. Finally, the polymers, within the type of resin (a mass of chemical compound chains) attend a plastics manufacturing plant, wherever additives offer the plastic the specified properties. Then it's molded or shaped into a plastic product.

13.8. Resin

In polymer chemistry and materials science, resin is a solid or highly viscous substance of plant or synthetic origin that is typically convertible into polymers. Resins are usually mixtures of organic compounds. Ion exchange resin has exchangeable cation or anions

There are two types of resin

1. Cation-exchange resin
2. Anion exchange resin

13.8.1. Cation-exchange Resin

The cation exchange method removes the hardness of water but induces acidity in it, which is further removed in the next stage of treatment of water by passing this acidic water through an anion exchange process. Formula: R–H acidic

Reaction:

$$R–H + M^+ = R–M + H^+.$$

13.8.2. Anion-exchange Resin

Often these are styrene–divinylbenzene copolymer resins that have quaternary ammonium cations as an integral part of the resin matrix. Formula: NR4+OH–

Reaction:

$$NR_4+OH^- + HCl = NR_4+Cl- + H_2O.$$

13.8.3. Similarity of Cation and Anion Exchange Resin

Cation and anion exchange resins are both small, porous, plastic beads (approximately .5 mm diameter, which varies) that are fixed with a specific charge. This "fixed" charge cannot be removed and is part of the resin's crosslinked makeup or structure. Each resin bead must also contain a neutralizing counterion that is able to move in and out of the bead, which is replaced with an ion of similar charge during the process of ion exchange (when an aqueous solution is passed through the beads and the ion exchange occurs, removing the undesirable contaminant).

13.8.4. Difference of Cation and Anion Exchange Resin

The main difference between cation and anion resins is that one is positively charged (cation) and the other is negatively charged (anion). This makes them useful in removing different types of contaminants (which will also vary depending on their size and chemical composition). Cation and anion resin beads can be used together (mixed bed configuration) or in separate vessels (twin bed configuration), depending on the needs of the facility and if total removal of positively and negatively charged ions are required.

Although anion and cation exchange resins are the main two categories of resins used in ion exchange, there are four main types

1. Strong base anion
2. Weak base anion
3. Strong acid cation
4. Weak acid cation

Below is a general overview of what each of these types of resins are:

Strong base anion resins

Strong base anion (SBA) exchange resins are typically used for demineralization, dealkalization, and desilication, as well as removal of total organic carbon (TOC) or other organics depending on the type of resin. They are available in multiple varieties, each of which offer a unique set of benefits and constraints, but in general, SBA resins are strong enough to remove both strong and weak acids (including carbonic and silicic acid).

Weak base anion resins

Weak base anion (WBA) exchange resins are often paired with SBA units for demineralization applications as they only remove anions associated with stronger acids (like chloride and sulfate) and will not remove weak acids (like carbon dioxide and silica). This can be beneficial for facilities that wish to remove the stronger acids while leaving the weaker behind, but commonly, WBA and SBA are often used jointly to complete a more thorough demineralization process.

Strong acid cation resins

Strong acid cation (SAC) exchange resins are among the most widely used resins, especially for softening applications, as they are effective at complete removal of hardness ions such as magnesium (Mg+) or calcium (Ca2+). Certain varieties of SAC resins have also been developed for applications demanding removal of barium and radium from drinking water or other streams. SAC resins can be damaged by oxidants and fouled by iron or manganese, so care must be taken to avoid exposure of the resin to these materials.

Weak acid cation resins

Weak acid cation (WAC) exchange resins remove cations associated with alkalinity (temporary hardness) and are used for demineralization and dealkalization applications. Additionally, WAC resins tend to have relatively high oxidation resistance and mechanical durability, making them a good choice for streams containing oxidants such as hydrogen peroxide and chlorine.

13.8.5.   Uses of Resin

- Resins are used to replace the magnesium and calcium ions found in hard water with sodium ions in water softening

- It is used to remove poisonous (e.g. copper) and hazardous metal (e.g. lead or cadmium) ions from solution, replacing them with more innocuous ions, such as sodium and potassium in water purification

- Ion exchange resins are used in organic synthesis, e.g. for esterification and hydrolysis.

- Resins are used in the manufacture of fruit juices such as orange and cranberry juice, where they are used to remove bitter-tasting components and so improve the flavor.

- Ion-exchange resins are used in the manufacturing of sugar from various sources.

- Resins are used in the manufacturing of pharmaceuticals, not only for catalyzing certain reactions, but also for isolating and purifying pharmaceutical active ingredients.

14. Instrumentation

14.1. Gas Chromatography (GC)

Gas Chromatography (GC or GLC) is a commonly used analytic technique in many research and industrial laboratories for quality control as well as identification and quantitation of compounds in a mixture. GC is also a frequently used technique in many environmental and forensic laboratories because it allows for the detection of very small quantities. A broad variety of samples can be analyzed as long as the compounds are sufficiently thermally stable and reasonably volatile.

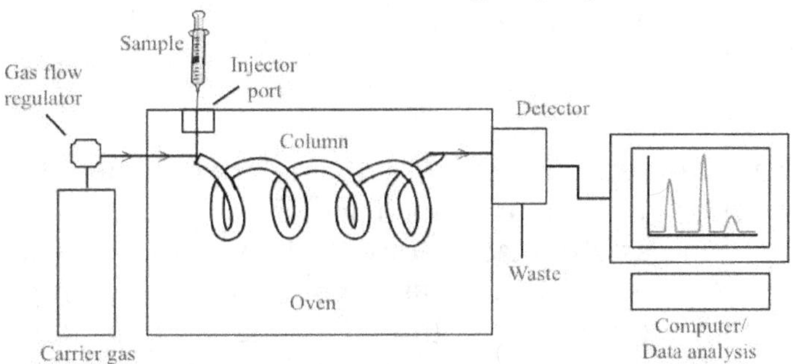

Sample Injection

A sample port is necessary for introducing the sample at the head of the column. Modern injection techniques often employ the use of heated sample ports through which the sample can be injected and vaporized in a near simultaneous fashion. A calibrated microsyringe is used to deliver a sample volume in the range of a few microliters through a rubber septum and into the vaporization chamber. Most separations require only a small fraction of the initial sample volume and a sample splitter is used to direct excess sample to waste. Commercial gas chromatographs often allow for both split and split less injections when alternating between packed columns and capillary columns. The vaporization chamber is typically heated 50

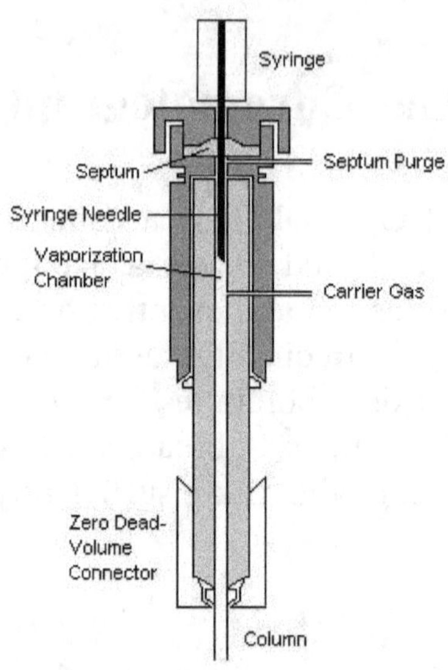

°C above the lowest boiling point of the sample and subsequently mixed with the carrier gas to transport the sample into the column.

Carrier Gas

The carrier gas plays an important role, and varies in the GC used. Carrier gas must be dry, free of oxygen and chemically inert mobile-phase employed in gas chromatography. Helium is most commonly used because it is safer than, but comparable to hydrogen in efficiency, has a larger range of flow rates and is compatible with many detectors. Nitrogen, argon, and hydrogen are also used depending upon the desired performance and the detector being used. Both hydrogen and helium, which are commonly used on most traditional detectors such as Flame Ionization(FID), thermal conductivity (TCD) and Electron capture (ECD), provide a shorter analysis time and lower elution temperatures of the sample due to higher flow rates and low molecular weight. For instance, hydrogen or helium as the carrier gas gives the highest sensitivity with TCD because the difference in thermal conductivity between the organic vapor and hydrogen/helium is greater than other carrier gas. Other detectors such as mass spectroscopy, uses nitrogen or argon which has a much better advantage than hydrogen or helium due to their higher molecular weights, in which improve vacuum pump efficiency.

Column Oven

The thermostatted oven serves to control the temperature of the column within a few tenths of a degree to conduct precise work. The oven can be operated in two manners: isothermal programming or temperature programming. In isothermal programming, the temperature of the column is held constant throughout the entire separation. The optimum column temperature for isothermal operation is about the middle point of the boiling range of the sample. However, isothermal programming works best only if the boiling point range of the sample is narrow. If a low isothermal column temperature is used with a wide boiling point range, the low boiling fractions are well resolved but the high boiling fractions are slow to elute with extensive band broadening. If the temperature is increased closer to the boiling points of the higher boiling components, the higher boiling components elute as sharp peaks but the lower boiling components elute so quickly there is no separation.

Open Tubular Columns and Packed Columns

Open tubular columns, which are also known as capillary columns, come in two basic forms. The first is a wall-coated open tubular (WCOT) column and the second type is a support-coated open tubular (SCOT) column. WCOT columns are capillary tubes that have a thin later of the stationary phase coated along the column walls. In SCOT columns, the column walls are first coated with a thin layer (about 30 micrometers thick) of adsorbent solid, such as diatomaceous earth, a material which consists of single-celled, sea-plant skeletons. The adsorbent solid is then treated with the liquid stationary phase. While SCOT columns are capable of holding a greater volume of stationary phase than a WCOT column due to its greater sample capacity, WCOT columns still have greater column efficiencies.

Detectors

1. Mass Spectrometer (GC/MS)

Many GC instruments are coupled with a mass spectrometer, which is a very good combination. The GC separates the compounds from each other, while the mass spectrometer helps to identify them based on their fragmentation pattern.

2. Flame Ionization Detector (FID)

This detector is very sensitive towards organic molecules (10-12 g/s = 1 pg/s, linear range: 106-107), but relative insensitive for a few small molecules i.e., N_2, NO_x, H_2S, CO, CO_2, H_2O. If proper amounts of hydrogen/air are mixed, the combustion does not afford any or very few ions resulting in a low background signal. If other carbon containing components, are introduced to this stream, cations will be produced in the effluent stream. The more carbon atoms are in the molecule, the more fragments are formed and the more sensitive the detector is for this compound. Unfortunately, there is no direct relationship between the number of carbon atoms and the size of the signal. As a result, the individual response factors for each compound have to be experimentally determined for each instrument. Due to the fact that the sample is burnt (pyrolysis), this technique is not suitable for preparative GC. In addition, several gases are usually required to operate a FID: hydrogen, oxygen (or compressed air), and a carrier gas.

3. Thermal Conductivity Detector (TCD)

This detector is less sensitive than the FID (10-5-10-6 g/s, linear range: 103-104), but is well suited for preparative applications, because the sample is not destroyed. The detection is based on the comparison of two gas streams, one containing only the carrier gas, the other one containing the carrier gas and the compound. Naturally, a carrier gas with a high thermal conductivity i.e., helium or hydrogen is used in order to maximize the temperature difference (and therefore the difference in resistance) between two filaments (=

thin tungsten wires). The large surface-to-mass ratio permits a fast equilibration to a steady state. The temperature difference between the reference and the sample cell filaments is monitored by a Wheatstone bridge circuit (the student learnt about this circuitry in physics!).

4. Electron Capture Detector (ECD)

This detector consists of a cavity that contains two electrodes and a radiation source that emits -radiation (i.e., 63Ni, 3H). The collision between electrons and the carrier gas (methane plus an inert gas) produces a plasma-containing electrons and positive ions. If a compound is present that contains electronegative atoms, those electrons will be "captured" to form negative ions and the rate of electron collection will decrease. The detector is extremely selective for compounds with atoms of high electron affinity (10-14 g/s), but has a relatively small linear range (~102-103). This detector is frequently used in the analysis of chlorinated compounds i.e., pesticides (herbicides, insecticides), polychlorinated biphenyls, etc. for which it exhibits a very high sensitivity.

Recorder

The recorder should be generally 10 mv (full scale) fitted with a fast response pen (1 sec or less). The recorder should be connected with a series of good quality resistances connected across the input to attenuate the large signals. An integrator may be a good addition.

Applications

- GC analysis is used to calculate the content of a chemical product, for example in assuring the quality of products in the chemical industry; or measuring toxic substances in soil, air or water.
- Gas chromatography is used in the analysis of:

    (a) air-borne pollutants
    (b) performance-enhancing drugs in athlete's urine samples

(c) oil spills

(d) essential oils in perfume preparation

- GC is very accurate if used properly and can measure picomoles of a substance in a 1 ml liquid sample, or parts-per-billion concentrations in gaseous samples.
- Gas Chromatography is used extensively in forensic science. Disciplines as diverse as solid drug dose (pre-consumption form) identification and quantification, arson investigation, paint chip analysis, and toxicology cases, employ GC to identify and quantify various biological specimens and crime-scene evidence.

Limitations

- Compound to be analyzed should be stable under GC operation conditions.
- They should have a vapor pressure significantly greater than zero.
- Typically, the compounds analyzed are less than 1,000 Da, because it is difficult to vaporize larger compounds.
- The samples are also required to be salt-free; they should not contain ions.
- Very minute amounts of a substance can be measured, but it is often required that the sample must be measured in comparison to a sample containing the pure, suspected substance known as a reference standard.

14.2. High Performance Liquid Chromatography (HPLC)

High Performance Liquid Chromatography (HPLC) is a form of column chromatography that pumps a sample mixture or analyte in a solvent (known as the mobile phase) at high pressure through a column with chromatographic packing material (stationary phase). The sample is carried by a moving carrier gas stream of helium or nitrogen. HPLC has the ability to separate, and identify compounds that are present in any sample that can be dissolved in a liquid in trace concentrations as low as parts per trillion. Because of this versatility, HPLC is used in a variety of industrial and scientific applications, such as pharmaceutical, environmental, forensics, and chemicals.

Sample retention time will vary depending on the interaction between the stationary phase, the molecules being analyzed, and the solvent, or solvents used. As the sample passes through the column it interacts between the two phases at different rate, primarily due to different polarities in the analytes. Analytes that have the least amount of interaction with the stationary phase or the most amount of interaction with the mobile phase will exit the column faster.

Types of HPLC

1. Normal Phase HPLC

This method separates analytes on the basis of polarity. NP-HPLC uses polar stationary phase and non-polar mobile phase. Therefore, the stationary phase is usually silica and typical mobile phases are hexane, methylene chloride, chloroform, diethyl ether, and mixtures of these.

Polar samples are thus retained on the polar surface of the column packing longer than less polar materials.

2. Reverse Phase HPLC

The stationary phase is nonpolar (hydrophobic) in nature, while the mobile phase is a polar liquid, such as mixtures of water and methanol or acetonitrile. It works on the principle of hydrophobic interactions hence the more nonpolar the material is, the longer it will be retained.

3. Size-exclusion HPLC

The column is filled with material having precisely controlled pore sizes, and the particles are separated according to its their molecular size. Larger molecules are rapidly washed through the column; smaller molecules penetrate inside the porous of the packing particles and elute later.

4. Ion-Exchange HPLC

The stationary phase has an ionically charged surface of opposite charge to the sample ions. This technique is used almost exclusively with ionic or ionizable samples.

The stronger the charge on the sample, the stronger it will be attracted to the ionic surface and thus, the longer it will take to elute. The mobile phase is an aqueous buffer, where both pH and ionic strength are used to control elution time.

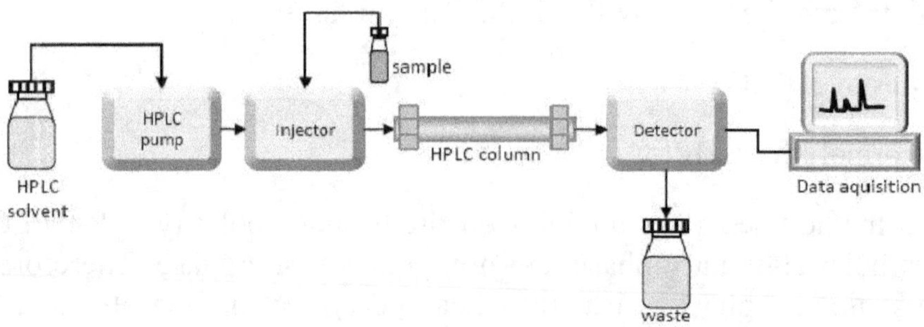

As shown in the schematic diagram in Figure above, HPLC instrumentation includes a pump, injector, column, detector and integrator or acquisition and display system. The heart of the system is the column where separation occurs.

1. Solvent Reservoir

Mobile phase contents are contained in a glass reservoir. The mobile phase, or solvent, in HPLC is usually a mixture of polar and non-polar liquid components whose respective concentrations are varied depending on the composition of the sample.

2. Pump

A pump aspirates the mobile phase from the solvent reservoir and forces it through the system's column and detector. Depending on a number of factors including column dimensions, particle size of the stationary phase, the flow rate and composition of the mobile phase, operating pressures of up to 42000 kPa (about 6000 psi) can be generated.

3. Sample Injector

The injector can be a single injection or an automated injection system. An injector for an HPLC system should provide injection of the liquid sample within the range of 0.1-100 mL of volume with high reproducibility and under high pressure (up to 4000 psi).

4. Columns

Columns are usually made of polished stainless steel, are between 50 and 300 mm long and have an internal diameter of between 2 and 5 mm. They are commonly filled with a stationary phase with a particle size of 3–10 μm.

Columns with internal diameters of less than 2 mm are often referred to as microbore columns. Ideally the temperature of the mobile phase and the column should be kept constant during an analysis.

5. Detector

The HPLC detector, located at the end of the column detect the analytes as they elute from the chromatographic column. Commonly used detectors are UV-spectroscopy, fluorescence, mass-spectrometric and electrochemical detectors.

6. Data Collection Devices

Signals from the detector may be collected on chart recorders or electronic integrators that vary in complexity and in their ability to process, store and reprocess chromatographic data. The computer integrates the response of the detector to each component and places it into a chromatograph that is easy to read and interpret.

Applications of High-Performance Liquid Chromatography (HPLC)

The HPLC has developed into a universally applicable method so that it finds its use in almost all areas of chemistry, biochemistry, and pharmacy.

- Analysis of drugs

- Analysis of synthetic polymers
- Analysis of pollutants in environmental analytics
- Determination of drugs in biological matrices
- Isolation of valuable products
- Product purity and quality control of industrial products and fine chemicals
- Separation and purification of biopolymers such as enzymes or nucleic acids
- Water purification
- Pre-concentration of trace components
- Ligand-exchange chromatography
- Ion-exchange chromatography of proteins
- High-pH anion-exchange chromatography of carbohydrates and oligosaccharides

Limitations

- Cost: Despite its advantages, HPLC can be costly, requiring large quantities of expensive organics.
- Complexity
- HPLC does have low sensitivity for certain compounds, and some cannot be detected as they are irreversibly adsorbed.
- Volatile substances are better separated by gas chromatography.

14.3. Thin Layer Chromatography (TLC)

Thin layer chromatography uses a thin glass plate coated with either aluminum oxide or silica gel as the solid phase. The mobile phase is a solvent chosen according to the properties of the components in the mixture. The principle of TLC is the distribution of a compound between a solid fixed phase (the thin layer) applied to a glass or plastic plate and a liquid mobile phase (eluting solvent) that is moving over the solid phase. A small amount of a compound or mixture is applied to a starting point just above the bottom of TLC plate.

The plate is then developed in the developing chamber that has a shallow pool of solvent just below the level at which the sample was applied. The solvent is drawn up through the particles on the plate through the capillary action, and as the solvent moves over the mixture each compound will either remain with the solid phase or dissolve in the solvent and move up the plate. Whether the compound moves up the plate or stays behind depend on the physical properties of that individual compound and thus depend on its molecular structure, especially functional groups. The solubility rule " Like Dissolves Like" is followed. The more similar the physical properties of the compound to the mobile phase, the longer it will stay in the mobile phase. The mobile phase will carry the most soluble compounds the furthest up the TLC plate. The compounds that are less soluble in the mobile phase and have a higher affinity to the particles on the TLC plate will stay behind 1.

On completion of the separation, each component appears as spots separated vertically. Each spot has a retention factor (Rf) expressed as:

Rf = dist. travelled by sample / dist. travelled by solvent

The factors affecting retardation factor are the solvent system, amount of material spotted, absorbent and temperature. TLC is one of the fastest, least expensive, simplest and easiest chromatography technique.

Plate preparation

 TLC plates are usually commercially available, with standard particle size ranges to improve reproducibility. They are prepared by mixing the adsorbent, such as silica gel, with a small amount of inert binder like calcium sulfate (gypsum) and water. This mixture is spread as thick slurry on an unreactive carrier sheet, usually glass, thick aluminum foil, or plastic. The resultant plate is dried and activated by heating in an oven for thirty minutes at 110 °C. The thickness of the adsorbent layer is typically around 0.1- 0.25 mm for analytical purposes and around 0.5- 2.0 mm for preparative TLC.

Spotting the plate

The thin end of the spotter is placed in the dilute solution; the solution will rise up in the capillary (capillary forces). Touch the plate briefly at the start line. Allow the solvent to evaporate and spot at the same place again. This way you will get a concentrated and small spot. Try to avoid spotting too much material, because this will deteriorate the quality of the separation considerably ('tailing'). The spots should be far enough away from the edges and from each other as well. If possible, you should spot the compound or mixture together with the starting materials and possible intermediates on the plate.

Location of spots

The position of various solutes separated by TLC can be located by various methods. Colored substances can be seen directly when viewed against stationary phase, while colorless substances can be detected only by making them visible by making use of some spraying agent, which produces colored areas in the region which they occupy.

Development solvents

The choice of a suitable solvent depends upon: Nature of substance, and adsorbent used on the plate. A development solvent should be such that, does not react chemically with the substances in the mixture under examination. Carcinogenic solvents (benzene etc) or environmentally dangerous solvents (dichloromethane etc) should always be avoided. Solvent systems range from non-polar to polar solvents. Non-polar solvents are generally used, as highly polar solvents cause the adsorption of any component of the solvent mixture. Commonly used development solvents are petroleum ether, carbon tetrachloride, pyridine, glycol, glycerol, diethyl ether, formamide, methanol, ethanol, acetone, and n-propanol.

Mobile Phase

For silica gel chromatography, the mobile phase is an organic solvent or mixture of organic solvents. As the mobile phase moves pass the surface of the silica gel it transports the analyte pass the particles of the stationary phase. However, the analyte molecules are only free to move with the solvent if they are not bound to the surface of the silica gel. Thus, the fraction of the time that the analyte is bound to the surface of the silica gel relative to the time it spends in solution determines the retention factor of the analyte. The ability of an analyte to bind to the surface of the silica gel in the presence of a particular solvent or mixture of solvents can be viewed as the sum of two competitive interactions. First, polar groups in the solvent can compete with the analyte for binding sites on the surface of the silica gel. Therefore, if a highly polar solvent is used, it will interact strongly with the surface of the silica gel and will leave few sites on the stationary phase free to bind with the analyte. The analyte will, therefore, move quickly pass the stationary phase. Similarly, polar groups in the solvent can interact strongly with polar functionality in the analyte and prevent interaction of the analyte with the surface of the silica gel.

This effect also leads to rapid movement of the analyte pass the stationary phase. The polarity of a solvent to be used for chromatography can be evaluated by examining the dielectric constant (å) and dipole moment (ä) of the solvent. The larger these two numbers, the more polar is the solvent. In addition, the hydrogen bonding ability of the solvent must also be considered. For example methanol is a strong hydrogen bond donor and will severely inhibit the ability of all but the most polar analytes to bind the surface of the silica gel.

Developing a Plate

A TLC plate can be developed in a beaker or closed jar. Place a small amount of solvent (mobile phase) in the container. A small spot of solution containing the sample is applied to a plate, about one centimeter from the base. The plate is then dipped in to a suitable solvent, such as hexane or ethyl acetate, and placed in a sealed container. The solvent moves up the plate by capillary action and meets the sample mixture, which is dissolved and is carried up the plate by the solvent.

Different compounds in the sample mixture travel at different rates due to the differences in their attraction to the stationary phase, and because of differences in solubility in the solvent. By changing the solvent, or perhaps using a mixture, the separation of components (measured by the Rf value) can be adjusted. The solvent level has to be below the starting line of the TLC, otherwise the spots will dissolve away. The lower edge of the plate is then dipped in a solvent. The solvent (eluent) travels up the matrix by capillarity, moving the components of the samples at various rates because of their different degrees of interaction with the matrix (stationary phase) and solubility in the developing solvent. Non-polar solvents will force non-polar compounds to the top of the plate, because the compounds dissolve well and do not interact with the polar stationary phase. Allow the solvent to travel up the plate until ~1 cm from the top. Take the plate out and mark the solvent front immediately. Do not allow the solvent to run over the edge of the plate. Next, let the solvent evaporate completely.

The TLC Experiment:

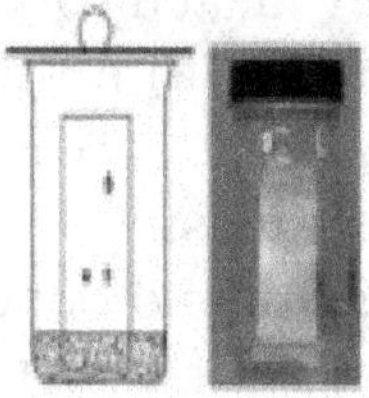

Lc chamber for development
with a lid or a closed jar

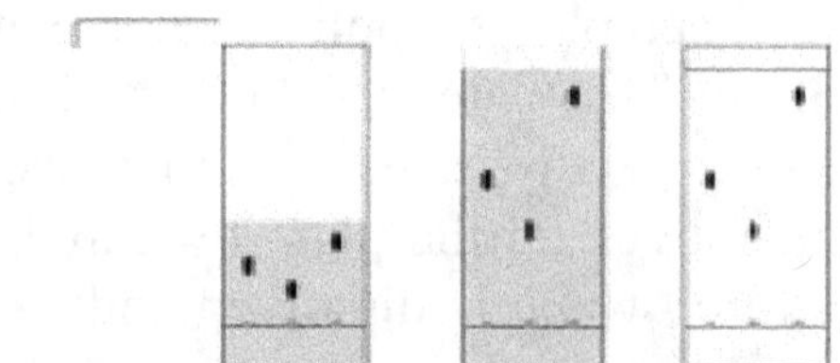

After ~5 Min   After ~10 Min   After Drying

Visualization

When the solvent front has moved to within about 1 cm of the top end of the adsorbent (after 15 to 45 minutes), the plate should be removed from the developing chamber, the position of the solvent front marked, and the solvent allowed to evaporate. If the components of the sample are colored, they can be observed directly. If not, they can sometimes be visualized by shining ultraviolet light on the plate or by allowing the plate to stand for a few minutes in a closed container in which the atmosphere is saturated with iodine vapor. Sometimes the spots can be visualized by spraying the plate with a reagent that will react with one or more of the components of the sample.

Analysis

The components, visible as separated spots, are identified by comparing the distances they have traveled with those of the known reference materials. Measure the distance of the start line to the solvent front. Then measure the distance of center of the spot to the start line. Divide the distance the solvent moved by the distance the individual spot moved. The resulting ratio is called Rf-value. As the chemicals being separated may be colorless, several methods exist to visualize the spots. Often a small amount of a fluorescent compound, usually manganese-activated zinc silicate, is added to the adsorbent that allows the visualization of spots under a blacklight (UV254). The adsorbent layer will thus fluoresce light green by itself, but spots of analyte quench this fluorescence, Iodine vapors are a general unspecific color reagent, Specific color reagents exist into which the TLC plate is dipped or which are sprayed onto the plate. Once visible, the Rf value, or retention factor, of each spot can be determined by dividing the distance traveled by the product by the total distance traveled by the solvent (the solvent front). These values depend on the solvent used, and the type of TLC plate, and are not physical constants.

Thin Layer Chromatography Applications

- The qualitative testing of various medicines such as sedatives, local anesthetics, anticonvulsant tranquilizers, analgesics, antihistamines, steroids, hypnotics is done by TLC.

- TLC is extremely useful in Biochemical analysis such as separation or isolation of biochemical metabolites from its blood plasma, urine, body fluids, serum, etc.
- Thin layer chromatography can be used to identify natural products like essential oils or volatile oil, fixed oil, glycosides, waxes, alkaloids, etc
- It is widely used in separating multicomponent pharmaceutical formulations.
- It is used to purify of any sample and direct comparison is done between the sample and the authentic sample
- It is used in the food industry, to separate and identify colors, sweetening agent, and preservatives
- It is used in the cosmetic industry.
- It is used to study if a reaction is complete.

14.4. Atomic Absorption Spectroscopy (AAS)

Atomic absorption spectrometry (AAS) detects elements in either liquid or solid samples through the application of characteristic wavelengths of electromagnetic radiation from a light source. Individual elements will absorb wavelengths differently, and these absorbances are measured against standards. In effect, AAS takes advantage of the different radiation wavelengths that are absorbed by different atoms.

In AAS, analytes are first atomized so that their characteristic wavelengths are emitted and recorded. Then, during excitation, electrons move up one energy level in their respective atoms when those atoms absorb a specific energy. As electrons return to their original energy state, they emit energy in the form of light. This light has a wavelength that is characteristic of the element. Depending on the light wavelength and its intensity, specific elements can be detected and their concentrations measured.

Instrumentation

Atomizer

In order for the sample to be analyzed, it must first be atomized. This is an extremely important step in AAS because it determines the sensitivity of the reading. The most effective atomizers create a large number of homogenous free atoms. There are many types of atomizers, but only two are commonly used: flame and electrothermal atomizers.

Flame atomizer

Flame atomizers are widely used for a multitude of reasons including their simplicity, low cost, and long length of time that they have been utilized. Flame atomizers accept an aerosol from a nebulizer into a flame that has enough energy to both volatilize and atomize the sample. When this happens, the sample is dried, vaporized, atomized, and ionized. Within this category of atomizers, there are many subcategories determined by the chemical composition of the flame. The composition of the flame is often determined based on the sample being analyzed. The flame itself should meet several requirements including sufficient energy, a long length, non-turbulent, and safe.

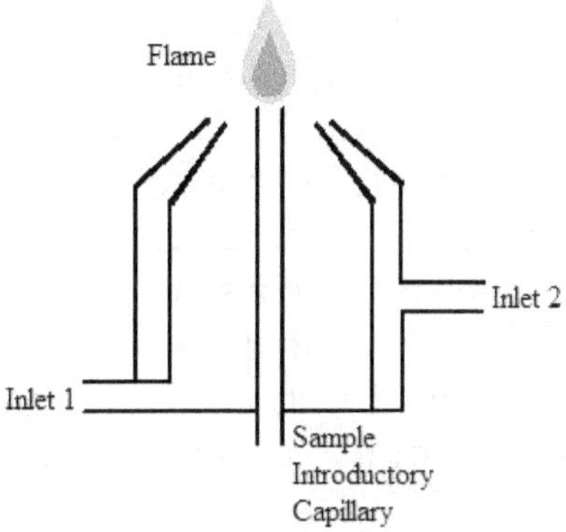

Electrothermal atomizer

Although electrothermal atomizers were developed before flame atomizers, they did not become popular until more recently due to improvements made to the detection level. They employ graphite tubes that increase temperature in a stepwise manner.

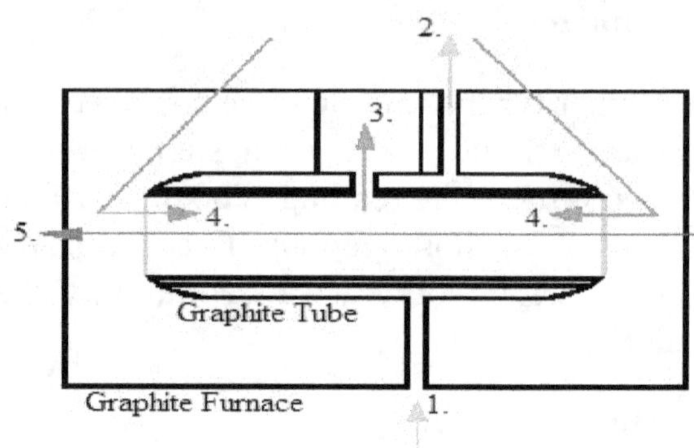

Electrothermal atomization first dries the sample and evaporates much of the solvent and impurities, then atomizes the sample, and then rises it to an extremely high temperature to clean the graphite tube. Some requirements for this form of atomization are the ability to maintain a constant temperature during atomization, have rapid atomization, hold a large volume of solution, and emit minimal radiation. Electrothermal atomization is much less harsh than the method of flame atomization.

Radiation source

The radiation source then irradiates the atomized sample. The sample absorbs some of the radiation, and the rest passes through the spectrometer to a detector. Radiation sources can be separated into two broad categories: line sources and continuum sources. Line sources excite the analyte and thus emit its own line spectrum. Hollow cathode lamps and electrodeless discharge lamps are the most commonly used examples of line sources. On the other hand, continuum sources have radiation that spreads out over a wider range of wavelengths. These sources are typically only used for background correction. Deuterium lamps and halogen lamps are often used for this purpose.

Spectrometer

Spectrometers are used to separate the different wavelengths of light before they pass to the detector. The spectrometer used in AAS can be either single-beam or double-beam. Single-beam spectrometers only require radiation that passes directly through the atomized sample, while double-beam spectrometers, as implied by the

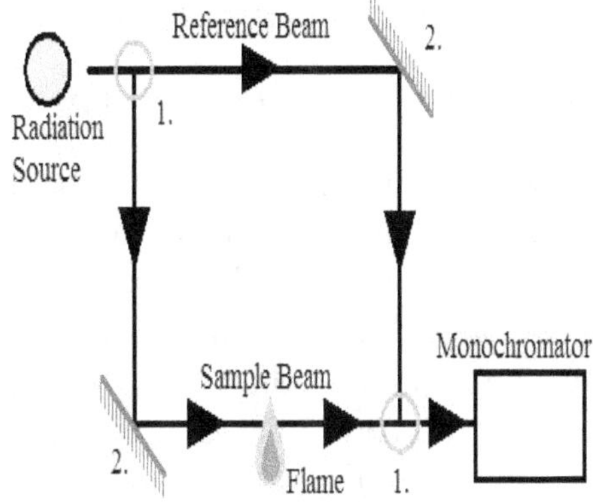

name, require two beams of light; one that passes directly through the sample, and one that does not pass through the sample at all. (Insert diagrams) The single-beam spectrometers have less optical components and therefore suffer less radiation loss. Double-beam monochromators have more optical components, but they are also more stable over time because they can compensate for changes more readily.

14.5. UV-Visible Spectrophotometer

Ultraviolet-visible (UV-Vis) spectrophotometry is a technique used to measure light absorbance across the ultraviolet and visible ranges of the electromagnetic spectrum. When incident light strikes matter it can either be absorbed, reflected, or transmitted. The absorbance of radiation in the UV-Vis range causes atomic excitation, which refers to the transition of molecules from a low-energy ground state to an excited state.

Before an atom can change excitation states, it must absorb sufficient levels of radiation for electrons to move into higher molecular orbits. Shorter bandgaps typically correlate to absorption of shorter wavelengths of light. The energy required for molecules to undergo these transitions, therefore, are electrochemically-specific. A UV-Vis spectrophotometer can use this principle to quantify the analytes in a sample based on their absorption characteristics.

Principle of UV spectroscopy

UV spectroscopy obeys the Beer-Lambert law, which states that: when a beam of monochromatic light is passed through a solution of an absorbing substance, the rate of decrease of intensity of radiation with thickness of the absorbing solution is proportional to the incident radiation as well as the concentration of the solution. The expression of Beer-Lambert law is-

$A = \log (I_0/I) = Ecl$

Where, A = absorbance

I_0 = intensity of light incident upon sample cell

I = intensity of light leaving sample cell

C = molar concentration of solute

L = length of sample cell (cm.)

E = molar absorptivity

From the Beer-Lambert law it is clear that greater the number of molecules capable of absorbing light of a given wavelength, the greater the extent of light absorption. This is the basic principle of UV spectroscopy.

Instrumentation

Instrumentation and working of the UV spectrometers can be studied simultaneously. Most of the modern UV spectrometers consist of the following   parts-

Light Source

Tungsten filament lamps and Hydrogen-Deuterium lamps are most widely used and suitable light source as they cover the whole UV region. Tungsten filament lamps are rich in red radiations; more specifically they emit the radiations of 375 nm, while the intensity of Hydrogen-Deuterium lamps falls below 375 nm.

Monochromator

Monochromators generally composed of prisms and slits. The most of the spectrophotometers are double beam spectrophotometers. The radiation emitted from the primary source is dispersed with the help of rotating prisms. The various wavelengths of the light source which are separated by the prism are then selected by the slits such the rotation of the prism results in a series of continuously increasing wavelength to pass through the slits for recording purpose. The beam selected by the slit is monochromatic and further divided into two beams with the help of another prism.

Sample and reference cells

One of the two divided beams is passed through the sample solution and second beam is passé through the reference solution. Both sample and reference solution are contained in the cells. These cells are made of either silica or quartz. Glass can't be used for the cells as it also absorbs light in the UV region.

Detector

Generally two photocells serve the purpose of detector in UV spectroscopy. One of the photocell receives the beam from sample cell and second detector receives the beam from the reference. The intensity of the radiation from the reference cell is stronger than the beam of sample cell. This results in the generation of pulsating or alternating currents in the photocells.

Amplifier

The alternating current generated in the photocells is transferred to the amplifier. The amplifier is coupled to a small servometer. Generally current generated in the photocells is of very low intensity, the main purpose of amplifier is to amplify the signals many times so we can get clear and recordable signals.

Recording devices

Most of the time amplifier is coupled to a pen recorder which is connected to the computer. Computer stores all the data generated and produces the spectrum of the desired compound.

Applications of UV Spectroscopy

Detection of Impurities

- It is one of the best methods for determination of impurities in organic molecules.
- Additional peaks can be observed due to impurities in the sample and it can be compared with that of standard raw material.
- By also measuring the absorbance at specific wavelength, the impurities can be detected.

Structure elucidation of organic compounds

- It is useful in the structure elucidation of organic molecules, such as in detecting the presence or absence of unsaturation, the presence of hetero atoms.
- UV absorption spectroscopy can be used for the quantitative determination of compounds that absorb UV radiation.
- UV absorption spectroscopy can characterize those types of compounds which absorbs UV radiation thus used in qualitative determination of compounds. Identification is done by comparing the absorption spectrum with the spectra of known compounds.
- This technique is used to detect the presence or absence of functional group in the compound. Absence of a band at particular wavelength regarded as an evidence for absence of particular group.
- Kinetics of reaction can also be studied using UV spectroscopy. The UV radiation is passed through the reaction cell and the absorbance changes can be observed.
- Many drugs are either in the form of raw material or in the form of formulation. They can be assayed by making a

suitable solution of the drug in a solvent and measuring the absorbance at specific wavelength.

- Molecular weights of compounds can be measured spectrophotometrically by preparing the suitable derivatives of these compounds.
- UV spectrophotometer may be used as a detector for HPLC.

14.6. Infrared Spectroscopy (IR)

Infrared (IR) spectroscopy or vibrational spectroscopy is an analytical technique that takes advantage of the vibrational transitions of a molecule. It is one of the most common and widely used spectroscopic techniques employed mainly by inorganic and organic chemists due to its usefulness in determining structures of compounds and identifying them. The method or technique of infrared spectroscopy is conducted with an instrument called an infrared spectrometer to produce an infrared spectrum.

Infrared Spectroscopy is the analysis of infrared light interacting with a molecule.

The portion of the infrared region most useful for analysis of organic compounds have a wavelength range from 2,500 to 16,000 nm

Photon energies associated with this part of the infrared (from 1 to 15 kcal/mole) are not large enough to excite electrons, but may induce vibrational excitation of covalently bonded atoms and groups.

It is known that in addition to the facile rotation of groups about single bonds, molecules experience a wide variety of vibrational motions, characteristic of their component atoms. Consequently, virtually all organic compounds will absorb infrared radiation that corresponds in energy to these vibrations.

Infrared spectrometers, similar in principle to other spectrometer, permit chemists to obtain absorption spectra of compounds that are a unique reflection of their molecular structure.

The fundamental measurement obtained in infrared spectroscopy is an infrared spectrum, which is a plot of measured infrared intensity versus wavelength (or frequency) of light. IR Spectroscopy measures the vibrations of atoms, and based on this it is possible to determine the functional groups. Generally, stronger bonds and light atoms will vibrate at a high stretching frequency (wavenumber).

Instrumentation

The main parts of IR spectrometer are as follows:

1. radiation source
2. sample cells and sampling of substances
3. Monochromators
4. detectors
5. recorder

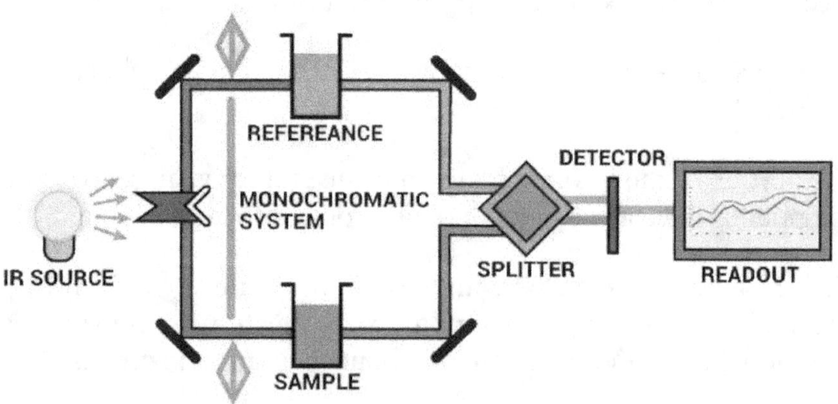

IR radiation sources

IR instruments require a source of radiant energy which emit IR radiation which must be steady, intense enough for detection and extend over the desired wavelength. Various sources of IR radiations are as follows.

a) Nernst glower

b) Incandescent lamp
c) Mercury arc
d) Tungsten lamp
e) Glober source
f) Nichrome wire

Sample cells and sampling of substances

IR spectroscopy has been used for the characterization of solid, liquid or gas samples.

1. Various techniques are used for preparing solid samples such as pressed pellet technique, solid run in solution, solid films, mull technique etc.
2. Samples can be held using a liquid sample cell made of alkali halides. Aqueous solvents cannot be used as they will dissolve alkali halides. Only organic solvents like chloroform can be used.
3. Sampling of gas is similar to the sampling of liquids.

Monochromators

Various types of monochromators are prism, gratings and filters. Prisms are made of Potassium bromide, Sodium chloride or Caesium iodide. Filters are made up of Lithium Fluoride and Diffraction gratings are made up of alkali halides.

Detectors

Detectors are used to measure the intensity of unabsorbed infrared radiation. Detectors like thermocouples, Bolometers, thermisters, Golay cell, and pyro-electric detectors are used.

Recorders

Recorders are used to record the IR spectrum.

Applications of Infrared (IR) Spectroscopy

It has been of great significance to scientific researchers in many fields such as:

- Protein characterization
- Nanoscale semiconductor analysis and
- Space exploration.
- Analysis of gaseous, liquid or solid samples
- Identification of compounds
- Quantitative analysis
- Information regarding functional groups of molecules and constitution of molecules can be deduced from IR spectrum
- To know about interaction among molecules

14.7. Fourier Transform Infrared Spectroscopy (FTIR)

The FTIR instrument relies upon interferences of various frequencies of light to produce a spectrum. It has a source, sample, two mirrors, a laser reference, and detector, but the assembly of components also include a beamsplitter and the two strategic mirrors that function as an interferometer.

The source energy strikes the beamsplitter and produces two beams of roughly the same intensity. One beam strikes the fixed mirror and returns to the beamsplitter. The other beam goes to the moving mirror. The motion of the moving mirror makes the total pathlength variable versus that taken by the fixed mirror beam. When these two beams meet up again at the beamsplitter, they recombine, and the difference in their path lengths create constructive and destructive interference, an interferogram.

The recombined beam passes through the sample. The sample absorbs all the wavelengths characteristic of the its spectrum and then subtracts specific wavelengths from the interferogram. The detector now reports variation in energy-versus-time for all wavelengths simultaneously. A laser beam is superimposed to provide a reference for the operation of the instrument.

A mathematical function known as a Fourier transform is used to convert the intensity-versus-time spectrum into an intensity-versus-frequency spectrum.

Instrumentation

It has same instrumentation as like IR Spectrophotometer. The main parts of FTIR spectrometer are as follows:

1. radiation source
2. sample cells and sampling of substances
3. Monochromators
4. detectors
5. recorder

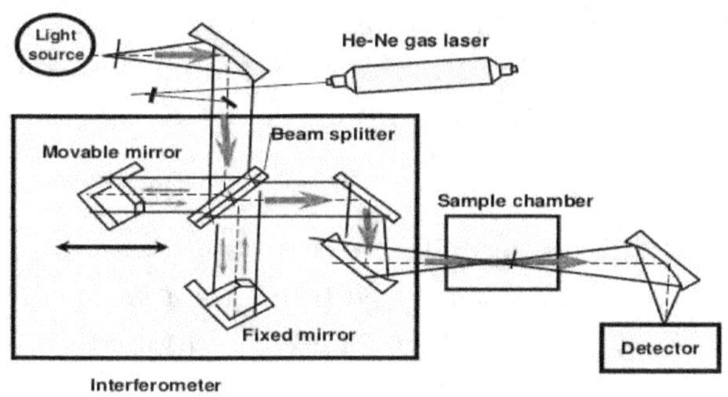

Applications of FTIR

Some of the more common applications are:

- Quality verification of incoming/outgoing materials
- Deformulation of polymers, rubbers, and other materials through thermogravimetric infra-red (TGA-IR) or gas chromatography infra-red (GC-IR) analysis
- Microanalysis of small sections of materials to identify contaminants
- Analysis of thin films and coatings
- Monitoring of automotive or smokestack emissions
- Failure analysis

14.8. Nuclear Magnetic Resonance (NMR)

Nuclear magnetic resonance spectroscopy, most commonly known as NMR spectroscopy or magnetic resonance spectroscopy (MRS), is a spectroscopic technique to observe local magnetic fields around atomic nuclei. It is a spectroscopy technique which is based on the absorption of electromagnetic radiation in the radio frequency region 4 to 900 MHz by nuclei of the atoms.

Of all the spectroscopic methods, it is the only one for which a complete analysis and interpretation of the entire spectrum is normally expected.

The sample is placed in a magnetic field and the NMR signal is produced by excitation of the nuclei sample with radio waves into nuclear magnetic resonance, which is detected with sensitive radio receivers.

The intramolecular magnetic field around an atom in a molecule changes the resonance frequency, thus giving access to details of the electronic structure of a molecule and its individual functional groups.

As the fields are unique or highly characteristic to individual compounds, NMR spectroscopy is the definitive method to identify monomolecular organic compounds. Besides identification, NMR spectroscopy provides detailed information about the structure, dynamics, reaction state, and chemical environment of molecules.

The most common types of NMR are proton and carbon-13 NMR spectroscopy, but it is applicable to any kind of sample that contains nuclei possessing spin.

NMR Spectroscopy Instrumentation

This instrument consists of nine major parts. They are discussed below:

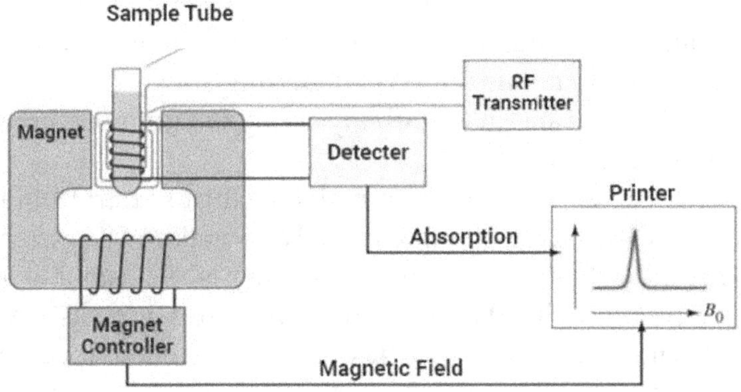

Sample holder: It is a glass tube which is 8.5 cm long and 0.3 cm in diameter.

Magnetic coils: Magnetic coil generates magnetic field whenever current flows through it

Permanent magnet: It helps in providing a homogenous magnetic field at 60 – 100 MHZ

Sweep generator: Modifies the strength of the magnetic field which is already applied.

Radiofrequency transmitter: It produces a powerful but short pulse of the radio waves.

Radiofrequency: It helps in detecting receiver radio frequencies.

RF detector: It helps in determining unabsorbed radio frequencies.

Recorder: It records the NMR signals which are received by the RF detector.

Readout system: A computer that records the data.

NMR Spectroscopy Applications

- NMR spectroscopy is a Spectroscopy technique used by chemists and biochemists to investigate the properties of organic molecules, although it is applicable to any kind of sample that contains nuclei possessing spin.
- The NMR can quantitatively analyze mixtures containing known compounds.
- NMR can either be used to match against spectral libraries or to infer the basic structure directly for unknown compounds.
- Once the basic structure is known, NMR can be used to determine molecular conformation in solutions as well as in studying physical properties at the molecular level such as conformational exchange, phase changes, solubility, and diffusion.

14.9. Total Organic Carbon (TOC)

Total Organic Carbon (TOC) is a measure of the total amount of carbon in organic compounds in pure water and aqueous systems. TOC is a valued, analytical technique that is applied by organizations and labs to determine how suitable a solution is for their processes. Unless it's ultrapure, water will naturally contain some organic compounds, understanding how much is key.

TOC has become an important parameter used to monitor overall levels of organic compounds present. This has happened despite the lack of any direct quantitative correlation between total organic carbon and the total concentration of organic compounds present and reflects the importance of having an easy-to-measure, general indicator of the approximate level of organic contamination.

It also reflects the appeal of a parameter which has a name which sounds more fundamental than it is! In many cases, the TOC is used as an on-going monitor of change or lack of change in organic content.

Measurement of TOC

When completing TOC analysis, the following is measured:

• TC – Total Carbon

• TIC – Total Inorganic Carbon

• POC – Purgeable Organic Carbon

• NPOC – Non-Purgeable Organic Carbon

• DOC – Dissolved Organic Carbon

• NDOC – Non-Dissolved Organic Carbon

To calculate TOC, you can subtract the total amount of inorganic carbon from total carbon found. Alternatively, you can add Purgeable and Non-Purgeable Organic Carbon, or Dissolved and Non-Dissolved Organic Carbon. As sums, they look like:

TOC = TC - TIC

TOC = POC + NPOC

TOC = DOC + NDOC

14.10.   Karl Fischer Titrator

Karl Fischer titration is a titration method that uses volumetric or coulometric titration to determine the quantity of water present in a given analyte. This method for quantitative chemical analysis was developed by the German chemist Karl Fischer in the year 1935, Today, specialized titrators (known as Karl Fischer titrators) are available to carry out such titrations.

Principle of Karl Fischer Titration

The principle of Karl Fischer titration is based on the oxidation reaction between iodine and sulfur dioxide. Water reacts with iodine and sulfur dioxide to form sulfur dioxide and hydrogen iodide. An endpoint is reached when all the water is consumed. The chemical equation for the reaction between sulfur dioxide, iodine, and water (which is employed during Karl Fischer titration) is provided below.

$$I_2 + SO_2 + H_2O \rightarrow 2HI + SO_3$$

The Karl Fischer titration experiment can be performed in two different methods. They are:

Volumetric determination: This technique is suitable to determine water content down to 1% of water. The sample is dissolved in KF methanol and the iodine is added to KF Reagent. The endpoint is detected potentiometrically.

Coulometric determination: The endpoint is detected in this experiment electrochemically. Iodine required for KF reaction is obtained by anodic oxidation of iodide from solution.

Karl Fischer Titration Instrumentation

Drying tube, sample injection cap, electrode analysis, Drain cook, a cathode chamber, detection electrode, rotor, anode chamber, KF reagent.

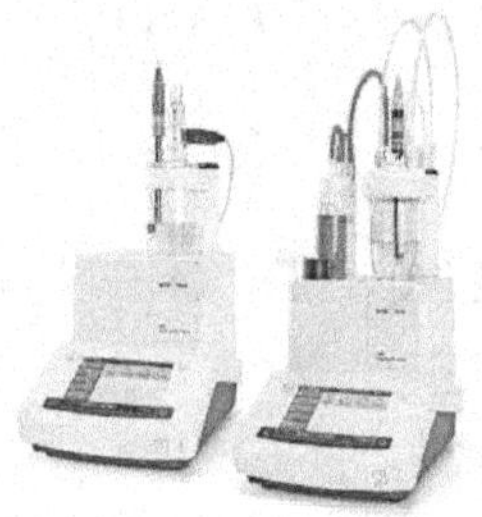

Ingredients of KF reagent: Iodine, Buffer (Imidazole), sulfur dioxide, solvent (methanol).

Karl Fischer Titration Applications

- It is used in technical products such as plastics, oils, gases.
- It is used in pharmaceutical products.
- It is used in cosmetic products.
- It is used in the industry.

Advantages of Karl Fischer Titration

- It is fitted for determining water in gases, liquids and solids.
- The coulometric titrator helps in detecting free water, dissolved water, and emulsified water.
- It is a swift process which demands a minimal amount of sample preparation.
- Extremely accurate method.

Limitations of Karl Fischer Titration

- It is a destructive technique.
- The solvent consumption is high as the manual volumetric titration demands reloading during each determination.
- Coulometric titration is fitted only for samples that contain a small amount of water.
- Coulometric titration takes extremely long periods to determine.

14.11.   pH meter

pH is a measurable parameter between the values of 0 and 14, provided the concentration of the solution does not exceed 1M. Solutions with a pH<7 are acidic, whereas those with a pH>7 are alkaline.

A pH meter is a scientific instrument that measures the hydrogen-ion activity in water-based solutions, indicating its acidity or basicity expressed as pH.

Instrumentation of pH meter

Fundamentally, a pH meter consists of a voltmeter attached to a pH-responsive electrode and a reference (unvarying) electrode. The pH-responsive electrode is usually glass, and the reference is usually a mercury–mercurous chloride (calomel) electrode, although a silver–silver chloride electrode is sometimes used. When the two electrodes are immersed in a solution, they act as a battery. The glass electrode develops an electric 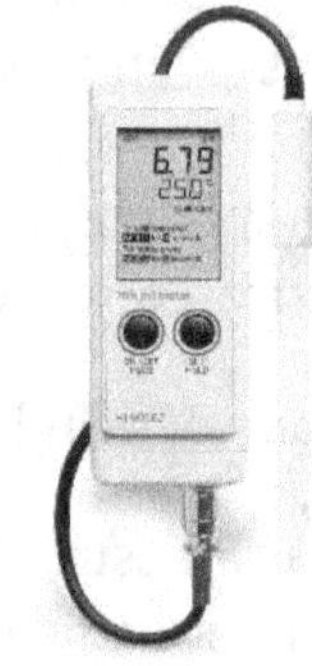 potential (charge) that is directly related to the hydrogen-ion activity in the solution (59.2 millivolts per pH unit at 25 °C [77 °F]), and the voltmeter measures the potential difference between the glass and reference electrodes.

14.12. Conductivity Meter

A conductivity meter measures the amount of electrical current or conductance in a solution. Conductivity is useful in determining the overall health of a natural water body. It is also a way to measure changes in wastewater procedures at water treatment plants. Conductivity meters are common in any water treatment or monitoring situation, as well as in environmental laboratories.

Conductivity is the electrical current in a solution, but that value depends on the liquid's ionic strength. It also relies on which ions are present, in what concentration and in what form, such as what state of oxidation or mobility the ions are in. Ions carry a negative or positive electrical charge: anions are negative and cations are positive. In natural water bodies, the ions that contribute to high conductivity result from dissolved minerals and salts. 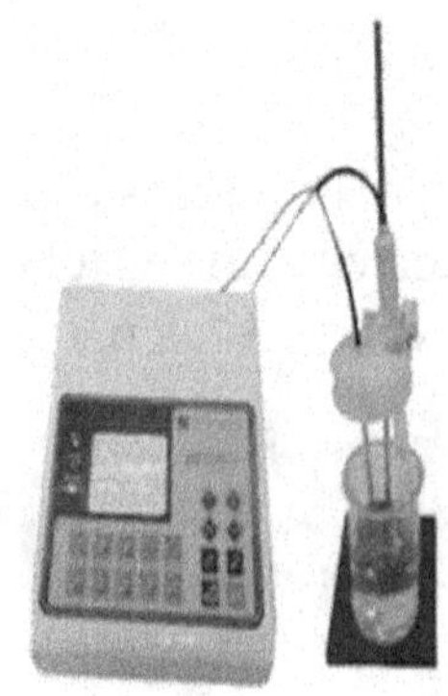

Instrumentation of conductivity meter

The meter is equipped with a probe, usually handheld, for field or on-site measurements. After the probe is placed in the liquid to be measured, the meter applies voltage between two electrodes inside the probe. Electrical resistance from the solution causes a drop in voltage, which is read by the meter. The meter converts this reading to milli- or micromhos or milli- or microSiemens per centimeter. This value indicates the total dissolved solids. Total dissolved solids is the amount of solids that can pass through a glass-fiber filter.

14.13.   Centrifuge Machine

A centrifuge is a laboratory device that is used for the separation of fluids, gas or liquid, based on density. Separation is achieved by spinning a vessel containing material at high speed; the centrifugal force pushes heavier materials to the outside of the vessel. This apparatus is found in most laboratories from academic to clinical to research and used to purify cells, subcellular organelles, viruses, proteins, and nucleic acids. There are multiple types of centrifuge, which can be classified by intended use or by rotor design. From the large floor variety to the micro-centrifuge, there are many varieties available for the researcher.

Centrifuge Categories:

Benchtop Centrifuges are a broad class of centrifuges characterized by their small bench space footprint. Depending on the research need, a variety of different aspects can be considered. Maximum speed in RCFs can range from as low as a few hundred to over 50,000 x g. Tube volumes can range from under 1 mL (such as with PCR tubes) to a few liters. Different types of rotors such as fixed angle, swinging bucket, and continuous flow are also typically interchangeable

Refrigerated Benchtop Centrifuges are compact instruments ideal for centrifugation of samples that may be temperature sensitive, such as live cells, animals or proteins. Many feature interchangeable rotors and adaptors to accommodate a wide range of sample volumes from under 1 mL to a few liters. Speeds can also vary, and some models can reach up to 60,000 x g

Clinical Benchtop Centrifuges are compact, low-speed centrifuges ideal for the separation of whole blood components, such as serum, plasma, buffy coat, red blood cells, as well as other bodily fluids. Their speeds may range between around 200 rpm to 6,000 rpm. Most clinical centrifuges can accommodate common blood draw tubes, but be sure to check with each vendor for specific tube sizes or tube adaptors.

Micro centrifuges are staple instruments in many research laboratories that generally accommodate small tube volumes such as 2 mL, 1.5 mL, 0.5 mL and PCR tubes. Microcentrifuges for routine laboratory procedures typically spin at speeds up to 16,000 x g, while more specialized instruments can reach speeds up to 30,000 x g. In addition, manufacturers may also offer interchangeable rotors and tube adaptors.

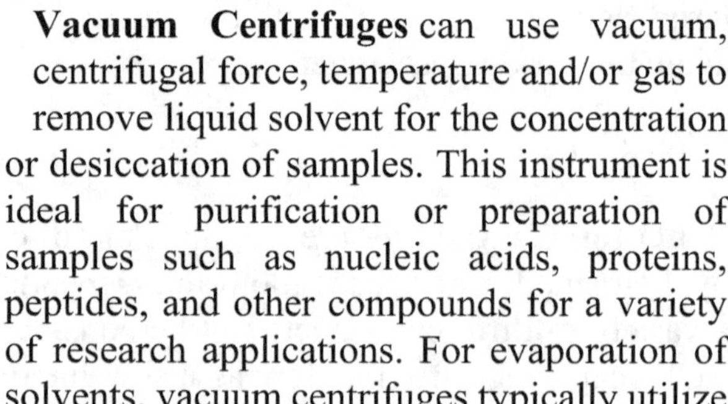

Vacuum Centrifuges can use vacuum, centrifugal force, temperature and/or gas to remove liquid solvent for the concentration or desiccation of samples. This instrument is ideal for purification or preparation of samples such as nucleic acids, proteins, peptides, and other compounds for a variety of research applications. For evaporation of solvents, vacuum centrifuges typically utilize built in heating systems.

14.14. **Electronic Balance**

Electronic balances have become standard equipment for chemistry laboratories. They allow the user to quickly and accurately measure the mass of a substance to a level of accuracy impossible for traditional balances to achieve. This is especially important in experiments that require precise amounts of each substance to achieve the desired results. The popularity of the electronic balance is also due to its extreme ease of use for any skill level.

How to use

Place the electronic balance on a flat, stable surface indoors. The precision of the balance relies on minute factors and wind, shaky surfaces, or similar forces will cause the readings to be inaccurate.

Press the "ON" button and wait for the balance to show zeroes on the digital screen.

Use tongs or gloves to place the empty container you will use for the substance to be measured on the balance platform. Fingerprints and other greases from your hands add mass and must be avoided for accurate measurements.

Press the "Tare" or "Zero" button to automatically deduct the weight of the container from future calculations. The digital display will show zero again, indicating that the container's mass is stored in the balance's memory.

Carefully add the substance to the container. Ideally this is done with the container still on the platform, but it may be removed if necessary. Avoid placing the container on surfaces that may have substances which will add mass to the container such as powders or grease.

Place the container with the substance back on the balance platform if necessary and record the mass as indicated by the digital display.

15. Water Treatment Plant (WTP)

Water Treatment Plant we call it shortly WTP. It is a concept where it covers all types of water treatment solution, such as nd so on. Water Treatment Plant is, collectively, the industrial-scale processes that make water more acceptable for an end-use, which may be used for drinking, industry or medicine.

Water Treatment is the procedure of eliminating undesirable chemicals, biological contaminants, suspended solids and gases from polluted water. The objective is to produce water fit for a specific purpose. Most water is disinfected for human consumption, but water purification may also be designed for a variety of other purposes, including fulfilling the requirements of medical, pharmacological, chemical and industrial applications. The methods of purification are depending of water contamination. For purification generally use physical processes such as filtration, sedimentation, and distillation; biological processes such as slow sand filters or biologically active carbon; chemical processes such as flocculation and chlorination and the use of electromagnetic radiation such as ultraviolet light. The Purifying water may reduce the concentration of particulate matter including suspended particles, parasites, bacteria, algae, viruses, fungi, as well as reducing the amount of a range of dissolved and particulate material derived from the surfaces that come from runoff due to rain.

15.1. Impurities

Each impurity carries its own risks to chemical and biological research, not to mention the detrimental effect they cause to the quality of pure water. Here we discuss the 8 main types of water contaminants, and how they can be prevented.

Microorganisms

Bacteria, algae and fungi all regularly interfere with sterile research applications. Bacteria can adversely influence cell and tissue culture by competing at enzyme-active sites on substrates.

If free-floating bacteria form biofilms on surfaces, they can be extremely difficult to remove. These biofilms can grow for several years, spontaneously releasing bursts of bacteria, along with their associated endotoxins and nucleases.

These nucleases then break down DNA and RNA in samples, and the endotoxins will have a negative effect on the growth and function of cells.

Viruses

Viruses – referred to as non-living nucleic acids – adversely affect tissue and cell growth. They're extremely small, with most of them falling between 0.01 – 0.3 microns, and they can survive for long periods of time. Once they've been spotted in water, they should be removed as soon as possible.

Pyrogens

For mammalian cell cultures, and the preparation of solutions or devices that will later have contact with humans and other mammals, it's crucial that the water used is pyrogen-free.

The most significant component of pyrogens – a form of endotoxin – is lipopolysaccharides (LPS), which is derived from Gram-negative bacteria walls. If LPS gets into the blood or spinal fluid, it can be toxic and cause a fever.

Dissolved Inorganic Ions

Silicates, chlorides, calcium, fluorides, magnesium, phosphates, bicarbonates, sulphates, nitrates and ferrous compounds are all forms of dissolved inorganic ions.

The instability in water caused by these ions will negatively influence chemical and biological reactions. Results include the formation of protein-protein and protein-lipid interaction, altering enzymatic activity, and delaying the growth of cells and tissue.

Dissolved Organic Compounds

These are derived from animal and plant decay, in addition to any human activities that involve the introduction of alcohol, protein, pesticides, chloramine, herbicides or detergents into the environment.

Dissolved organic compounds interfere with high performance liquid chromatography (HPLC), gas chromatography and fluoroscopy.

Dissolved Gases

Water contains naturally dissolved carbon dioxide, nitrogen and oxygen, but these gases can alter the pH of lab water, which upsets the ionic balance. Concentrations of oxygen and nitrogen can affect the rate of biochemical reactions; and high concentration of dissolved gases can cause a bubble formation, which obstructs the flow through chromatography columns and micro-channels.

Dissolved carbon dioxide raises water acidity, reducing the capacity of ion exchange resins in DI systems.

Suspended Particles

When large suspended particles of clay, sand, silt or vegetation between $1 - 10\mu m$ are found in water, they cause turbidity and settle at the bottom. Suspended particles can foul reverse osmosis membranes, filters and chromatography columns, especially if the system stems from a reservoir or tank within the building.

Colloidal Particles

Colloidal particles are much smaller than suspended particles, at just $0.01 - 1.0\mu m$, and they don't settle. Colloidal particles regularly interfere with analytical techniques, and bypass ion exchange resins, which result in lower resistivity in DI water.

15.2. **Raw Water Treatment**

Raw water treatment plants are still being used throughout the United States. They typically consist of several steps in the treatment process. These include:

(1) Collection
(2) Screening and Straining
(3) Chemical Addition
(4) Coagulation and Flocculation
(5) Sedimentation and Clarification
(6) Filtration
(7) Disinfection
(8) Storage
(9) Distribution.

Let's examine these steps in more detail.

Collection – The source water for a municipal surface water treatment plant is typically a local river, lake, or reservoir. There must be a method to get this water to the water treatment plant. Quite often, a series of pumps and pipelines transport the water to the treatment plant. Sometimes, as is the case of San Angelo, water from a reservoir such as Twin Buttes can be transported to the water treatment plant via a river. Twin Buttes Reservoir is one of the water sources for San Angelo. The water is released into Lake Nasworthy where it is transported down the Concho River to the water treatment plant. At the water plant, large pumps are used to transfer the water up to the treatment facility. Treatment facilities are often engineered to utilize gravity water flow as much as possible to reduce pumping costs.

Many water treatment plants utilize water from more than one source. Blending groundwater with surface water is a method often used to improve the quality of the final product.

Screening and Straining – If you think about surface water sources, i.e., lakes, rivers, and reservoirs, you realize they contain varying amounts of suspended and dissolved materials. This material may include turbidity, color, taste, odor, microorganisms, fish, plants, trees, trash, etc. The material may be organic or inorganic, suspended or dissolved, inert or biologically active, and vary in size from colloidal to a tree trunk. Some of these larger items can impede equipment in the treatment process, such as a tree limb getting stuck in a water pump impeller. So the first process in conventional water treatment is to screen or strain out the larger items. This is often accomplished using a large metal screen, often called a bar-screen, which is placed in front of the water source intake. Large items are trapped on the screen as the water passes through it. These screens must routinely be raked or cleaned off.

Chemical Addition – Once the pre-screened source water is received into the treatment plant, chemicals are added to help make the suspended particles that are floating in the water clump together to form a heavier and larger gelatinous particle, often called floc. In this process, a chemical is added that reacts with the natural alkalinity in solution to form an insoluble precipitate. There are many different chemicals on the market that are used in this process. These chemicals are called. One of the most common that has been used for many years is aluminum sulfate, or alum. Some other very popular coagulants are ferrous sulfate, ferric chloride, sodium aluminate, activated silica, and compounds called polymers that are manufactured chemicals made up of repeated small units of low molecular weight combined into molecules with very large molecular weights. These polymers are classified as cationic polymers (positively charged), anionic polymers (negatively charged), and nonionic polymers (neutrally charged). Regardless of which coagulant or combination of coagulants is used, they must be mixed very well with the water before they can form a heavier floc.

Coagulation and Flocculation - A rapid mix unit is usually used where the coagulant is added to the water to provide a very quick and thorough mixing. The water mixing is then slowed to allow the water to come in contact with the forming floc and allow it to increase in size. The continued mixing must be gentle to allow the floc to grow and gain weight, but fast enough to keep it in suspension until you are ready for it to settle in the clarifiers. The process of adding a chemical to cause the suspended material to "clump" into larger particles is called flocculation or coagulation. The treatment unit where coagulation and flocculation are performed is called the "flocculator".

Sedimentation and Clarification – Once the flocculation process is complete, the water then passes over the weir in the flocculator and travels to the center of the clarifier, or sedimentation basin. Here, the water makes its way from the center of the clarifier to the saw tooth weir at the perimeter of the unit. As the water makes its way towards the weir, the large floc particles are allowed to settle out to the bottom of the clarifier. A rake continuously travels across the bottom of the clarifier and scrapes the settled floc to the center of the unit. Pumps are used to pull the settled "sludge" out of the clarifier and send it to a sedimentation / disposal pond. The water that passes over the weir is collected and transferred to the filters. The reason clarification occurs before filtration is so the majority of suspended material can be removed prior to filtration, which avoids overloading the filters and thus allowing much more water to be filtered before the filters must be backwashed.

Filtration – Clarified water enters the filters from the top. Gravity pulls the water down through the filters where it is collected in a drain system at the bottom of the unit. There are many different types of materials (media) used in filters. The most common being sand and gravel. Many conventional plants are now using granular activated carbon as the media of choice because it not only provides excellent mechanical filtration of particulate matter, but also removes organic compounds which can cause taste and odor problems.

Disinfection – Once the water has gone through the filtration process, it is about as clear and clean as it can get. However, there may still be bacteria and viruses remaining. To ensure these are destroyed, there must be a disinfection process employed. The most common disinfection process used in the United States is chlorination. Chlorine comes in many different forms including chlorine gas (most common), chlorine dioxide, hypochlorite (bleach), and others. Whichever method is used, chlorine is added to the water in an amount to ensure all microorganisms are destroyed. Water plants monitor the chlorine levels continuously and very carefully in the treated water. They must add enough chlorine to ensure thorough disinfection of the water, but avoid adding excesses that can cause taste and odor problems when delivered to the consumer.

Storage – Once the disinfection process is complete, the water is stored. Storage usually takes place in an underground storage tank called a "clear well", and also in elevated storage tanks that are visible around town. There must always be an ample supply of water available in the event of emergencies. These can include power outages, fires, floods, etc.

Distribution – So how does the water come out of your kitchen tap? The stored water is pushed through underground pipelines all over town in what is called a "distribution system". The distribution system consists of large water pumps at the treatment plant, overhead water storage tanks, large pipelines, smaller pipelines, fire hydrants, valves, and water meters in your front yard.

15.3. Advance Water Treatment

Water makes the world go round and is a critical part of life as we know it. Without water, very little could survive. Water helps all living things grow and survive in their natural environments. From serving up a pitcher of water at a restaurant to watering crops on a massive farm, water is used constantly. However, not all areas of the world are abundant in clean water. Some places even face droughts. All people need access to clean water in order to survive. Dirty water can kill plants, animals and make people very sick.

There are several processes that make up advanced water treatment. Together, these processes make water a useful, abundant commodity.

1. Boiler feed water treatment
2. Reverse osmosis
3. Membrane filtration
4. Water oxidation

15.3.1.   Boiler Feed Water Treatment

A boiler feed water treatment system is a system made up of several individual technologies that address your specific boiler feed water treatment needs.

Treating boiler feed water is essential for both high- and low-pressure boilers. Ensuring the correct treatment is implemented before problems such as fouling, scaling, and corrosion occur, will go a long way in avoiding costly replacements/upgrades down the line.

An efficient and well-designed boiler feed water treatment system should be able to:

- Efficiently treat boiler feed water and remove harmful impurities prior to entering the boiler
- Promote internal boiler chemistry control
- Maximize use of steam condensate
- Control return-line corrosion
- Avoid plant downtime and boiler failure
- Prolong equipment service life

Process of boiler feed water treatment system

As mentioned above, the exact components of a boiler feed water treatment system depend on the quality of water being drawn from in relation to the quality of water makeup needed for the specific boiler, but in general, a basic boiler feed water treatment system typically includes some type of:

- Filtration and ultrafiltration
- Ion exchange/softening
- Membrane processes such as reverse osmosis and nanofiltration
- Deaeration/degasification
- Coagulation/chemical precipitation

Depending on the impurities present in your water, any combination of these treatments might best suit your facility and make up your treatment system, and depending on the needs of your plant and process, these standard components are usually adequate. However, if your plant requires a system that provides a bit more customization, there might be some features or technologies you will need to add on.

15.3.2.   Reverse Osmosis

Reverse osmosis involves taking water from the ground and putting it through a process that removes all of the water's minerals and deionizes it so that it is safe for people to drink. Without this critical process, people would not be able to extract the harmful materials found in natural water and could become sick or die as a result. This process is used in desalinization, which is when ocean water is turned into clean, fresh water. Reverse osmosis helps remove the salt from ocean water leaving behind clean water. The world is running out of fresh and natural resources to use, and 97 percent of the water on the planet is salt water. Reverse osmosis can also help recycle water to make it clean and safe again, and also is used in wastewater treatments.

15.3.3.   Membrane Filtration

Membrane filtration is a streamlined process that helps create clean drinking water. This process is often used to improve food quality, as it helps separate particles from water to create other beverages such as beer, milk and juice. There are four different types of membrane filtration, including nanofiltration, ultra-filtration, reverse osmosis and microfiltration. A different type of filtration process is used for different sized particles. The particles found in salt water are the smallest, so reverse osmosis is used. However, the particles in river water might be larger, so microfiltration is used. Though water filtration is used for a variety of reasons, one is to help create beverages and dairy products in the food industry. This process helps concentrate and purify a variety of foods, from beverages such as beer and vegetable juice to dairy products such as yogurt and cheese. This process is used in several stages of food and beverage development so these products are safe to be sold and used.

15.3.4.   Water Oxidation

Water oxidation is used to break down water into two elements-hydrogen and oxygen. The process separates the water back into its original elements so that it can be used for other things. People and other living organisms need oxygen to live, so this process can be used anywhere where oxygen is readily needed, such as filling up oxygen tanks. Given that climate change and air pollution are currently harming the environment, people are looking for other sources of fuel, one of which is hydrogen. This treatment process helps provide water and hydrogen where it's needed to improve the environment as a whole.

15.3.5.   Mix Bed Polisher

Mixed bed ion exchange is an ion exchange process for polishing of demineralized water, meaning for removal of trace dissolved solids from water.

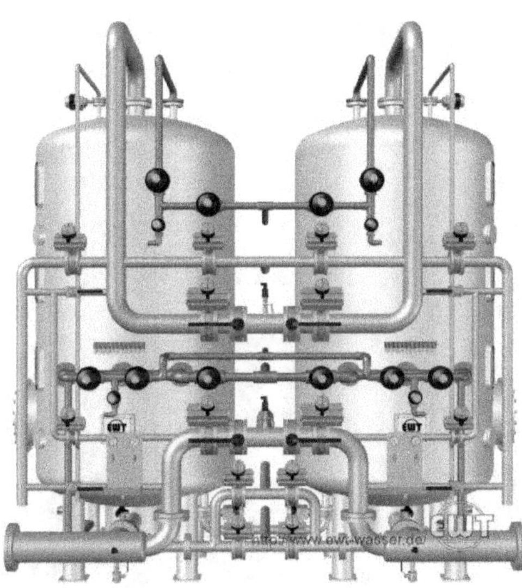

A mixed bed ion exchanger (also: mixed bed polisher, mixed bed filter) is a vessel filled with a mixture of cation exchange resin and anion exchange resin. During service, water flows through this resin mixture. Cations dissolved in the water are then exchanged for hydrogen ions (H+), while anions dissolved in the water are exchanged for hydroxide ions (OH-). Hydrogen ions and hydroxide ions react to water.

With increasing service life, the ion exchange resins deplete. Depleted mixed bed resins are regenerated, usually with both hydrochloric acid (HCl) and sodium hydroxide (NaOH). With each regeneration, potentially acidic or alkaline waste water is produced, which may need to be neutralized. In case of smaller mixed bed exchangers, the ion exchange resin is sometimes also discarded and exchanged once depleted, rather than regenerated.

Usually, a mixed bed ion exchanger is used either as a last polishing step downstream of another demineralization process, or as a working mixed bed for demineralization of already partly demineralized or low-TDS water

16. Effluent Treatment Plant (ETP)

Wastewater is water that has been used and must be treated before it is released into another body of water, so that it does not cause further pollution of water sources. Wastewater comes from a variety of sources. Everything that you flush down your toilet or rinse down the drain is wastewater. Rainwater and runoff, along with various pollutants, go down street gutters and eventually end up at a wastewater treatment facility. Wastewater can also come from agricultural and industrial sources. Some wastewaters are more difficult to treat than others; for example, industrial wastewater can be difficult to treat, whereas domestic wastewater is relatively easy to treat (though it is increasingly difficult to treat domestic waste, due to increased amounts of pharmaceuticals and personal care products that are found in domestic wastewater.

The objective of municipal and industrial waste water treatment is to extract pollutants, remove toxicants, neutralize coarse particles, kill pathogens so that quality of discharged water is improved to reach the permissible level of water to be discharged into water bodies or for agricultural land.

Treatment of water thus aims at reduction of BOD, COD, eutrophication etc. of receiving water bodies and prevention of bio-magnification of toxic substances in food chain.

Effluent Treatment plant consists of three steps

- Primary water treatment
- Secondary water treatment
- Tertiary water treatment

16.1. **Primary Water Treatment**

The primary level of treatment uses screens and settling tanks to remove the majority of solids. This step is extremely important, because solids make up approximately 35 percent of the pollutants that must be removed. The screens usually have openings of about 10 millimeters, which is small enough to remove sticks, garbage and other large materials from the wastewater. This material is removed and disposed of at the landfill.

The water is then put into settling tanks (or clarifiers), where it sits for several hours, allowing the sludge to settle and a scum to form on the top. The scum is then skimmed off the top, the sludge is removed from the bottom, and the partially treated wastewater moves on to the secondary treatment level. The primary treatment generally removes up to 50 percent of the Biological Oxygen Demand (BOD; these are substances that use up the oxygen in the water), around 90 percent of suspended solids, and up to 55 percent of fecal coliforms. While primary treatment removes a significant amount of harmful substances from wastewater, it is not enough to ensure that all harmful pollutants have been removed.

16.2. **Secondary Water Treatment**

Secondary treatment of wastewater uses bacteria to digest the remaining pollutants. This is accomplished by forcefully mixing the wastewater with bacteria and oxygen. The oxygen helps the bacteria to digest the pollutants faster. The water is then taken to settling tanks where the sludge again settles, leaving the water 90 to 95 percent free of pollutants. Secondary treatment removes about 85 to 90 percent of BOD and suspended solid, and about 90 to 99 percent of coliform bacteria.

Some treatment plants follow this with a sand filter, to remove additional pollutants. The water is then disinfected with chlorine, ozone, or ultraviolet light, and then discharged.

The sludge that is removed from the settling tanks and the scum that is skimmed off the top during the primary steps are treated separately from the water. Anaerobic bacteria (anaerobic bacteria do not require oxygen) feed off of the sludge for 10 to 20 days at temperatures around 38 degrees Celsius. This process decreases the odor and organic matter of the sludge, and creates a highly combustible gas of methane and carbon dioxide, which can be used as fuel to heat the treatment plant. Finally, the sludge is sent to a centrifuge, like the one shown in the picture below. A centrifuge is a machine that spins very quickly, forcing the liquid to separate from the solid. The liquid can then be processed with the wastewater and the solid is used as fertilizer on fields.

16.3. **Tertiary Water Treatment**

Tertiary (or advanced) treatment removes dissolved substances, such as color, metals, organic chemicals and nutrients like phosphorus and nitrogen. There are a number of physical, chemical and biological treatment processes that are used for tertiary treatment. One of the biological treatment processes is called Biological Nutrient Removal (BNR). This diagram shows the treatment steps that Saskatoon wastewater goes through.

Tertiary (or advanced) treatment removes dissolved substances, such as color, metals, organic chemicals and nutrients like phosphorus and nitrogen. There are a number of physical, chemical and biological treatment processes that are used for tertiary treatment. One of the biological treatment processes is called Biological Nutrient Removal (BNR).

For the tertiary treatment, the BNR process occurs in the bioreactors. The BNR process uses bacteria in different conditions in several tanks, to digest the contaminants in the water. The three tanks have unique environments, with different amounts of oxygen. As the water has passes through the three tanks, the phosphorus is removed and the ammonia is broken down into nitrate and nitrogen gas, which other bacterial processes can not do. The BNR process can remove over 90 percent of phosphates, while traditional processes remove much less than 90 percent. The water spends approximately nine hours in the bioreactors, before entering the secondary clarifier, which is a settling tank, where the bacteria-laden sludge settles to the bottom of the tank. In this treatment plant, wastewater first undergoes primary and secondary treatment. For the tertiary treatment, the BNR process occurs in the bioreactors. The BNR process uses bacteria in different conditions in several tanks, to digest the contaminants in the water. The three tanks have unique environments, with different amounts of oxygen. As the water has passes through the three tanks, the phosphorus is removed and the ammonia is broken down into nitrate and nitrogen gas, which other bacterial processes can not do. The BNR process can remove over 90 percent of phosphates, while traditional processes remove much less than 90 percent. The water spends approximately nine hours in the bioreactors, before entering the secondary clarifier, which is a settling tank, where the bacteria-laden sludge settles to the bottom of the tank.

17. Productivity Concept in Industry

People are engaged in various fields of economic activities like farms, factories, hospital, bank, schools, office is etc. To earn living by producing goods and services which is required by the community. The inter-relationship of all these economic activities is called an economic system which caters comfort and well-being of individuals. To produce goods and services resources in the form of men, machine, material and money are required. And the more efficient use of resources is ensured, no more goods and services will be produced. In fact, this efficient use of effective utilization of resources is truly proactivity, which is an essential element and successful strategy for the well-being of the individuals.

17.1. Definition of Productivity

Productivity is generally defined as a ration between output of benefits and input of resources. It implies how much input resources are required for production of certain amount of output or specifically output per unit of input. It means efficient use and effective utilization of different factor inputs. Productivity can be expressed as-

Productivity, P = Output of Benefits (Q) / Input of Resources (N)

17.2. Production and Productivity

Productivity is not production. The term "Productivity" is often confused with the term "Production". Many people think that greater the production, the greater the productivity. This is not necessarily true.

Production is concerned with the activity of producing goods and/or services while productivity is concerned with the efficient utilization of resources (input) in producing goods and services (output).

If viewed in quantitative terms, production is the quantity of output produced, while productivity is the ratio of the output produced to the inputs used.

For example, "X" enterprise produced 10000 radios by employing 50 workers at 8 hours per day 25 days. Then,

Production = 10 radios and Productivity, P = 10000 / (5*8*25) = 1 radio/man hour

Suppose in the next months, the same enterprise increases its production to 12000 radios by adding 10 additional workers at 8 hours per day for 25 days. Then,

Production = 12000 radios and Productivity, P = 12000 / (6*8*25) = 1 radio/man – hour

From the above example, it is clear that production of radio increased by 20% (from 10000 units to 12000 units) but productivity remains same.

17.3. Production, Productivity, Efficiency and Effectiveness

Production: IS concerned with the activity of producing goods and/or services.

Efficiency: Is the ratio of actual outputs produced to the standard outputs expected. For example, if output of and operator is 120 pieces/hr, while standard rate is 180 pieces/hr, the operator efficiency is said to be 120/180 = 0.6667 or 66.67 per cent.

Effectiveness: Is the degree of accomplishment of objectives. How well a set of result is accomplished reflects the effectiveness, whereas how well the resources are utilized to accomplish the results refers to the efficiency. Productivity is both efficiency and effectiveness.

Profitability: IS concerned with the efficient utilization of resources (input) in producing goods and/services (outputs).

1) Productivity = Output/Input

$$= \text{Doing Things Right (Efficiency)} + \text{Doing the Right Things (Effectiveness)}$$

2) Productivity = f (Efficiency, Effectiveness)
3) Productivity is better today than yesterday and better tomorrow than today. It is a continuous process.

17.4. **Measurement of Productivity**

Reasons to measure Productivity of an enterprise –

- ➢ To monitor performance
- ➢ To reveal problem area
- ➢ To appraise how well resources are utilized
- ➢ To improve productivity situation

Measurement of productivity depends upon two factors i.e. output indicators and input indicator.

17.4.1. **Output Indicators**

Output is production of goods and services by employing input resources.

Type of output:

1) Physical measure= Physical quantity, Type of physical product.
2) Value measure = Quantity * price = Value

Type of value measure:

a. Profit = Sale – expenditure
b. Gross value of production
c. Gross output: Includes:

       1. Sale – Change in stock;

2. Value of by product;

3. Income from service or other sources.

d. Value added: Gross output – Industrial and non-industrial cost.

Item of industrial cost: Cost of raw material used, fuel, power, electricity.

Non-Industrial Cost:

1) Printing and stationary,
2) Postage, telegraph and telephone cost,
3) Water charges, advertising and selling expenses (commission, banking, Insurance)
4) Consultancy service,
5) Accounting and auditing
6) Small repair maintenance
7) T.A., D.A. etc.

17.4.2.   Input Indicators

Input is resource or goods and service used as a means of production.

Input:

1) Manpower: Man day
2) Man Hour, etc.
3) Capital: Building & Instrument
4) Current Cost: Interest on Saving, Interest on Loan, Establishment Cost, Depreciation Cost, etc.
5) Non-Industrial Cost: Printing Cost, Telephone, Telegraph, Poster Cost, Advertisement Cost, Water Cost, Insurance Cost, Consultancy Cost, Audit Cost etc.
6) Energy: Fuel/Electricity

17.5. **Methods of Improving Productivity**

Productivity improvement depends upon better equipment utilization, elimination of wastage in all forms and conservation of energy. There are five possible ways in which productivity can be improved.

These are-

1) Reduce cost,
2) Manage growth,
3) Work smarter,
4) Pair down,
5) Work effectively

17.6. **Tools of Productivity Promotion**

1. Japanese 5S
2. KAIZEN
3. Suggestion Scheme
4. Benchmarking
5. QCC (Quality Control Circle)
6. TPM (Total Productive Maintenance)
7. JIT (Just in Time)

18. Popular Inventions in Chemistry

Chemistry is vastly intriguing. Had it not been for this wing of science, we tend to might have still been bereft of a transparent understanding of matter itself. Analysis within the field of chemistry alone has created North American countries tuned in to the atmosphere, the world and specifically, us. From Alchemy to chemistry, the science incorporates a history chemical analysis back to over 2500 years. Chemistry could be a branch of natural philosophy that is that the study of the composition, properties and behavior of matter. It's known as "the central science" because it relates to physics, earth science and biology. Allow us to, therefore, examine a number of the foremost important inventions during this howling science of Chemistry. The importance of inventions in chemistry is, therefore, necessary that we are forced to form this associate degree eleven purpose list.

Synthesis of Organic Compound

A German Chemist by the name of Friedrich Wohler provided the most important step within the field of Chemistry by synthesizing Urea for the primary time. In fact, this very important invention in Chemistry – creation of organic compound – refuted the 'belief or very important' that everyone living things were alive thanks to some "special vital force!" This pioneering step of conversion of ammonia cyanate into organic compound within the year 1828 is actually of mammoth historical significance as for the primary time associate degree compound was made from inorganic reactants. This large discovery light-emitting diode to the all necessary branch of chemistry.

Discovery of Atomic Number 8

'Fire Gas' or Oxygen was 1st discovered by Swedish caregiver Carl Wilhelm Scheele in 1772 however no documentation was printed relating to constant until 1777. it absolutely was a British spiritual leader chemist WHO is therefore given priority within the discovery as his findings were created legendary 1st in 1775. The invention of atomic number 8 thence is of prime importance within the timeline of

Chemistry. This eventually light-emitting diode to Lavoisier once and for all proving that atomic number 8 was a substance.

Atomic Theory

Atomic theory is outlined as a theory of the character of matter, that states that matter consists of distinct units known as atoms, as opposition the obsolete notion that matter might be divided into any indiscriminately little amount. John Dalton's atomic theory as printed within the year 1808 could be a important step within the evolution of chemistry. the issues in his theory were later corrected by physicist to provide North American country the Avogadro's Principle.

The entered the study of Chemical Structure in decennary: The study of molecular structure was delivered to the forefront within the 1850s by Friedrich August Kekule von Stradonitz. With the chemical structure of benzol being found out headway was potential in understanding the aromatic compounds, imperative eventually for each pure and applied chemistry as discovered within the consequent years.

Publication of Tabular Array of the Weather

Periodic Table is that the tabular show of chemical elements. Any student of chemistry begins his journey with this tabular array and thence the publication of constant is of utmost importance once one talks concerning the chronicles of Chemistry. Dmitri Mendeleyev is attributable with the primary widely known tabular array that he created public within the year 1869. Mendeleev's tabular array has over the years been developed and refined with the new inventions in chemistry.

Transformation of Chemicals by Electricity

Discoveries of many alkali and metallic element metals by Sir Humphry chemist tested that electricity transforms chemicals. Experiment with the employment of electrical piles to separate salt that was performed at that point by him is these days referred to as Electrolysis. many new metals were discovered as a result of these experiments like atomic number 11, potassium, magnesium, element and Ba.

Discovery that Atoms have Signatures of Sunshine

Gustav Gustav Robert Kirchhoff and Robert Bunsen discovered that every part absorbs or emits lightweight at specific wavelengths, manufacturing specific spectra. This was a very important discovery because it light-emitting diode to the understanding that colored flames might be differentiated by observing their emission spectra through a prism. This eventually assisted the fields of spectroscopic analysis and therefore the understanding of emission of electromagnetic radiation by heated objects.

Discovery of the Lepton

Johann Wilhelm Hittorf within the year 1869 discovered a glow emitted from a cathode that will increase in size with pressure. Eventually within the year 1896 British man of science J. J. Thomson conducted experiments to prove that the cathode rays were created of distinctive particles that he known as corpuscles. These particles were eventually named Electrons; imperative to several branches of science and our understanding of atomic theory and quantum physics.

Discovery of Inert Vaporish Elements

The discovery of the Noble gases- inert gas, krypton, and xenon, later isolated atomic number 2 determined within the spectrum of the sun and radon- is another milestone within the history of Chemistry. Scottish chemist Sir William Ramsay WHO discovered these gases was awarded the Nobel prize in Chemistry within the year 1904 for constant.

Van't Hoff's Discovery of Chemical Dynamics and Diffusion Pressure

The first winner of Nobel prize in Chemistry Jacobus Henricus van 't Hoff, Jr. helped the reason behind chemistry by discovering the laws of chemical dynamics and diffusion pressure in solutions. This helped in shaping the discipline of chemical science because it is these days. This discovery tested that terribly dilute solutions follow mathematical laws that closely match the laws describing the behavior of gases.

Penicillin

There's a good chance that penicillin saved your life at some point in time. Without it, a prick from a thorn or sore throat can easily turn fatal. Alexander Fleming gets the credit for penicillin when, in 1928, he observed how a mold growing on his Petri dishes suppressed the growth of nearby bacteria. But, despite his best efforts, he failed to extract any usable penicillin. Fleming gave up and the story of penicillin took a 10-year hiatus. Until in 1939, it took Australian pharmacologist Howard Florey and his team of chemists to figure out a way of purifying penicillin in useable quantities.
The team cobbled together a totally functional penicillin production plant from bathtubs, milk churns and bookshelves.

The Haber-bosch Process

Nitrogen plays a critical role in the biochemistry of every living being. It is also the most common gas in our atmosphere. But plants and animals can't extract it from the air. Consequently, a major limiting factor in agriculture has been the availability of nitrogen.
In 1910, German chemists Fritz Haber and Carl Bosch changed all this when they combined atmospheric nitrogen and hydrogen into ammonia. This, in turn, can be used as crop fertilizer, eventually filtering up the food chain to us.
Today, about 80 percent of the nitrogen in our body comes from the Haber-Bosch process, making this single chemical reaction probably the most important factor in the population explosion of the past 100 years.

Polythene the Accidental Invention

Most common plastic objects, from water pipes to food packaging and hard hats, are forms of polythene. The 80m tonnes of the stuff made each year is the result of two accidental discoveries. One occurred in 1898 when German chemist Hans von Pechmann while investigating something different, noticed a waxy substance at the bottom of his tubes. Along with his colleagues, he investigated and discovered that it was made up of very long molecular chains which they termed polymethylene. That's how polythene came into being.

Discovery of Radioactivity

Radioactivity was first discovered in 1896 by the French scientist Henri Becquerel, while he was working on phosphorescent material. It was initially thought to be similar to X-rays but further investigation by chemists and scientists like Becquerel, Ernest Rutherford, Paul Villard, Pierre Curie, Marie Curie, proved that this form of radioactivity was significantly more complicated.

Madam Curie first isolated Uranium from its ore which eventually led to the discovery of polonium and radium. Apart from nuclear power and nuclear weaponry, there remains a wide range of ways in which radioactive material and the radiation it gives off remain useful in the daily lives of people all over the world. Hospitals use radiation in a wide range of ways. X-ray, CT and Gamma radiation (PET) to produce detailed images of the human body.

19. Role of Chemistry in Human Life

Human body itself is formed of chemical compositions and therefore the setting needed for the human life to sustain is indivisible from the chemical composition of matters.

We all know our body is about 60% water, but then what composes the rest of it? Carbon, Hydrogen, Nitrogen and Oxygen. These elements compose 96% of the human body. Whereas the rest 4% is composed of about 60 elements. Some of these elements include calcium, phosphorus, potassium, and sulfur.

Most people consider chemistry as a boring and complicated, but this is untrue. It is because of chemistry many of our daily activities are achieved. Soaps, detergents, pills, plastics, clothes, food, colors, and many others are some of the products of chemistry.

Food

Food we eat is nothing but a mixture of various chemicals. From its production to cooking, chemistry plays a very important role. Consider tomatoes, they are produced in farms. Fertilizers and crop-protection chemicals like insecticides, pesticides etc., are used in farming to increase the production of tomatoes. Then ripped tomatoes are brought to food processing industries, where they are converted into a finished product like ketchup. After various stages of food processing different ingredients like flavoring agent, chemical additives are added based on chemistry. Finally, food products are passed on to Food safety and standards authority like the FDA in the US. This authority analyses the content of food by chemical tests and approves the food for consumer consumption

Detergents and soaps

We use detergents and soaps for cleaning, bathing, washing etc. They are a mixture of chemicals with cleaning properties. They are manufactured in chemical industries through saponification of fatty acids. Common chemicals used in soap industries are sodium hydroxide, potassium hydroxide, lauric acid, palmitic acid, oleic acid etc.

Medicine

Drugs are made of chemicals which are produced in pharmaceutical industries. The knowledge of chemistry is vital for pharmacists and doctors. Have you ever glance at the label of a medicine? If yes, then you have observed various chemical ingredients listed on the label. It is based on these ingredients medical practitioners decide a suitable pill for patients. The chemical nature of drugs also helps doctors to determine how drugs are going to interact with a patient's body. For example, antibiotics like ciprofloxacin and levofloxacin are dependent on renal functions. So, the doctor who prescribed such pills needs to be prudent for kidney patients. Chemicals are also used in sterilization, disinfection to kill microbes. Chemistry also helps pharmacists to understand biochemical mechanisms in a body.

Textiles

Raw materials used in textile industries are wool, silk, jute, cotton, flax, glass fiber, polyester, acrylic, nylon etc. These materials are transformed into usable finished products like clothes, bags, carpets, furniture, towels, flags, nets, balloons etc. During this transformation, raw materials are subjected to numerous chemical processes. Pre-treatment chemicals like cleaning and smoothing reagents are added to clean to fabric and smoothen it. Dyeing involves the application of fabric to dyes and pigments. Other chemical processes are bleaching, permanent press, desizing, scouring, printing, finishing. Chemists work to improve the quality of a product or involve in the development of new material.

Building & construction

Chemistry governs the performance of buildings. Building materials play a significant role in improving the performance of buildings. Coating chemicals like acrylics, silicones, urethanes are responsible for reflective roofs, which decreases the heat transfer. Polymers like polyurethane reduce the weight of buildings, which reduces the civil cost. Insulators like polyurethane foams, polystyrene foams decrease the heat leaks or in other words, improves the energy efficiency of the building. Polyethylene is a lightweight, flexible polymer which is used to create building piping. Polyethylene piping is easily curved and deformed to desired shapes. Vinyl tiles give shining, resilient flooring. Fillers like polystyrene beads lighten concrete without affecting the strength of concrete.

Paper and pulp industries

Over the last few decades, paper and pulp industries are responsible for negative impacts on the environment. Paper and pulp industries are facing grave challenges to meet environmental norms. Pollutants released from these industries are sulphur oxides, nitrogen oxides, carbon oxides, heavy metals (lead, cadmium, mercury), dioxins, furans, chlorates, chelating agents etc. To overcome this, industries are more focused on green chemistry to mitigate some of the environmental challenges. Green chemistry enables the researchers to design safer chemicals and products, to use renewable raw materials, converse the energy, to develop better catalyst etc.

Fuel

Petrol, diesel, LPG, CNG, kerosene, oils, hydrogen etc are all fuel produced from complex refining processes. Today's transportation (land, water, and air) is possible because of these fuels. These fuels are extracted from cruel oil found beneath the earth or oceans. Here petrochemistry plays an important role; it is a branch of chemistry which deals with the study of petrochemical processes.

Battery

Batteries are used in cars, cell phones, laptops, watches, flashlights, and many other power storage applications. Batteries work based on the principle of electrochemistry. The energy inside a battery is stored in the form of chemical energy, which converts into electric energy by electrochemical reaction.

Environmental protection

Chemistry is the central subject in the study of environmental conservation. All those pollutants and greenhouse gases nothing but hazardous chemicals. These pollutants destroy our precious environment, degrade the ozone layer, enter our food chain, and cause tumors and so forth. All these interactions of pollutant with the environment are chemical reactions. Hence, chemistry is vital to alleviate the environment and ourselves from these poisons.

Forensic

Forensic chemistry has made jobs of police officers a lot easier. Forensic helps to identify criminals by detecting chemical evidence left behind crime scenes. Chemical techniques used by forensic investigators are spectroscopy, chromatography, X-ray diffractometry, color tests, melting point analysis etc.

Nation's economy

Chemistry also contributes to the growth of a country. Chemical production increases the GDP of a nation. Chemical industries also generate employment.

Ourselves

We are a biological organism made up of various biochemicals like carbohydrates, proteins, vitamins, lipids etc. Our biological processes like digestion, respiration, cellular metabolism, reproduction, and many others are accomplished by biochemical reactions. In nutshell, we will not exist without chemistry.

20. Chemical Innovations That Will Change Our World

Nanopesticides

World population keeps growing. Some predictions suggest we will be almost 10 billion humans by 2050. Feeding that many people will require a huge increase in agricultural production, while keeping crops sustainable: minimizing the environmental impact in terms of land use, reducing the amount of water needed, and mitigating the contamination by agrochemicals such as fertilizers or pesticides. Unsurprisingly, nanotechnology is attracting quite a lot of attention beyond the pharma and health industries. Tailored nano-delivery systems could also become a great tool for farmers, as it would eventually allow them to tackle the main problems of conventional pesticides such as environmental contamination, bioaccumulation, and the huge increase in pest resistance. There are very few publications that carefully analyze the benefits—and risks—of so-called "nanoagrochemicals" against their conventional alternatives. In most cases, the increase in efficacy is quite limited. However, in some cases researchers have observed improvements by an order of magnitude under laboratory conditions. We still need a proper assessment of the efficacy of nanopesticides under field conditions. That is why some companies still investigate their potential, proving that there is still hope for this technology. Canadian Vive Crop is possibly the best example, selling products that have demonstrated better absorption and less environmental impact than their non-nano commercial alternatives. Moreover, this company recently received the approval of the U.S. Environmental Protection Agency to commercialize various nano-encapsulated insecticides and fungicides. Nanotechnology may not be the only ingredient to a successful new, more sustainable agriculture, but it will certainly lead to more sophisticated agrochemicals with a lower impact on the environment and human health.

Enantio-selective organocatalysis

Chemists have always been inspired by nature. A few years back, researchers dreamt of a new kind of catalysts that, like most natural enzymes, would not require the use of expensive metals. "Organocatalysis" was born in the late 1990s and it has not stopped growing ever since. According to Paolo Melchiorre, one of the leading experts in the field, organocatalysis was successful because "[It] was quite democratic, everyone could have access to it without needing expensive reagents or a glovebox, which allowed many young researchers to start their independent careers, and quickly assembled a community of international experts that become a great incubator of ideas for catalysis without metals," he explains.

Initially, some chemists criticized organocatalysis for not being as green as it claimed to be—it needed high catalyst loads and, moreover, it was hard to recover the catalyst after the reaction, which seem to go against the very definition of catalysis. However, Melchiorre points out how researchers have overcome most of these problems. He says that the original focus of organocatalysis was "to develop new methods rather than decreasing the catalyst loads."

Nevertheless, because chemists understood the industrial implications that lowering the catalyst amount could have, they crafted ways of creating chiral carbon–carbon bonds using just part per millions of organocatalysts. "This is still not comparable to metals, but the cost is significantly cheaper," he adds.

Chemists have also developed solutions to better recover the catalysts—Ben List immobilizes them on solid substrates like nylon, which is just one of the many possible answers. Melchiorre highlights how organocatalysis has seeded the chemical landscape and eventually sprung other fields, especially photoredox catalysis, which allows new types of transformations: "[David] MacMillan created the link between the two fields. Light activation enabled reactions such as the alkylation of aldehydes with enamines, which couldn't be done with classic organocatalytic methods." Many other fields have emerged from organocatalysis, and now industries have scaled-up asymmetric organocatalytic protocols to synthesis fine chemicals and drugs.

Solid-state batteries

Solid-state batteries were already envisioned in the 19th century by pioneer chemist Michael Faraday. However, their development never become a reality until quite recently. Now, important industries from a variety of sectors such as Bosch, Dyson, Toyota, and Intel are investing billions of dollars in this technology. John Goodenough, co-inventor of the now omnipresent lithium-ion batteries, recently unveiled a battery that uses glass as the electrolyte—proving that solid-state batteries are closer to market than ever. Compared to lithium-ion batteries that power our smartphones, tablets, and laptops, solid-state batteries are lighter, allow higher energy storage, and perform well at high temperatures. Moreover, unlike the electrolytes used in lithium-ion technology, solid-state electrolytes are not flammable, which could potentially avoid spontaneous fires and explosions, like the flames that darkened the launch of Samsung Galaxy Note 7 a few years back. However, the new technology is still very expensive.

As for many other applications, polymers may be the best and most economical solution. French transportation company Bolloré is already fabricating and commercializing polymer-based solid-state batteries, which they use mostly for network connected sensors.

According to polymer expert Tanja Junkers, "charge transporting polymers [are] truly fascinating—we have just yet seen the very beginning of what will be possible in [the] future." There is still a lot of research to be done, especially because solid-state battery components are so closely bound together that it is quite complicated to understand how each of them behaves.

Academics and industrial researchers are closely working together to develop better non-destructive, operando technologies—electron microscopy and nuclear magnetic resonance—to understand how solid-state batteries perform. For most uses, the technology will still need a few more years of development.

Flow chemistry

Chemistry is key in achieving some of the United Nation's Sustainable Development Goals (SDGs), a blueprint to attain a better and more sustainable future for all by the year 2030. Among them, flow chemistry, where reactions are run in a continuously flowing stream rather than in batch, is particularly critical for tackling SDG12: responsible consumption and production. Flow chemistry processes eventually minimize the risk of handling hazardous substances and increase productivity, both preventing harm and lowering the environmental impact. Although some people consider flow chemistry to be on a very early, small-scale laboratory stage, efficient industrial applications are increasingly common.

Back in 2015, chemists at MIT demonstrated the potential of flow chemistry to create tailored polymers that would be unattainable by classical batch techniques. According to the experts in the field, the flow process is quicker and simpler, yet more reliable, which is quite in line with the SDG goals.

More recent examples have even shown the potential of flow chemistry to withstand hazardous reagents such as organolithium compounds. Merck chemists achieved a 100kg-scale synthesis of a precursor for verubecestat, a phase III candidate to treat Alzheimer's disease. Other recent examples include the flow synthesis of ciprofloxacin, an essential antibiotic, and an automated flow system developed by Pfizer capable of analyzing up to 1500 reaction conditions a day, speeding up the discovery of optimal synthetic routes for both new and existing drugs.

Reactive extrusion

Along with flow chemistry comes reactive extrusion, a technique that allows chemical reactions to happen completely solvent-free. The elimination of potentially toxic solvents makes this process environmentally friendly. It creates however many engineering challenges as it would require a complete redesign of the industrial processes that are now in place. Although extrusion processes have been widely-used and investigated by polymer and material experts, it is only now that other chemists are starting to dig into their possibilities in the preparation of organic compounds. Classic extrusion methods involve grinding reagents in a ball mill, but more advanced extrusion technologies using screws could even allow these solvent-free reactions to operate in flow setups. Once again, the downside lays on effectively adapting the systems and scaling them up. In their labs, chemists have used ball mills to prepare several attractive products—amino acids, hydrazones, nitrones, and peptides—and have achieved some very classic organic reactions—Suzuki coupling, click chemistry—but the examples in reactive extrusion conditions beyond polymers remain quite elusive. However, the scarce exceptions show great promise. Biotech company Amgen reported the optimized synthesis of co-crystals with potential use in the treatment of chronic pain, which was also the first example of mechanochemical synthesis scaled-up to several hundred grams. Furthermore, scientists in the UK have used reactive extrusion to efficiently prepare deep eutectic solvents [11]—a class of ionic liquids that could become the new generation of green, non-flammable solvents. Both previous examples involve the formation of intramolecular interactions, but not the creation of new covalent bonds. However, chemists have recently reported the formation of **metal organic frameworks (MOFs)** and discrete metal complexes by screw extrusion, opening the door to new possibilities towards a cleaner and more sustainable solvent-free chemistry.

MOFs and porous materials for water harvesting

According to the United Nations (UN), water scarcity affects more than 40 % of the global population and is projected to rise. On top of that, three in ten people lack access to safely-managed drinking water services. Chemistry could bring a solution to this problem identified as SDG 6 "to change our world" using porous materials, particularly metal organic frameworks (MOFs). Porous materials like MOFs have a sponge-like chemical structure with microscopic spaces that can selectively trap molecules, from gases—hydrogen, methane, carbon dioxide, water—to more complex substances, such as drugs and enzymes. While some researchers were focusing on the uses of MOFs in drug delivery and gas purification, Omar Yaghi accidentally discovered their great potential in capturing water from the atmosphere. "When we were studying the trapping of post-combustion gases uptake into MOFs, we noticed that some MOFs exhibited a unique interaction with water molecules," explains Yaghi. Then, they wondered whether the same material "[could] be used to trap water from the atmosphere in arid climates, and then be released easily for collection." This technology is unique, because "it can harvest drinkable amounts of pure water from the dry desert air with no energy required other than the natural sunlight," says Yaghi. Just one kilogram of MOF could harvest 2.8 liters of water a day at a humidity level as low as 20 %. While working on higher capacity, potentially cheaper versions of the water-harvesting materials, Yaghi is "already partnering with companies to test their MOF water harvesters on an industrial scale." There are other porous materials with similar abilities such as silica-based and inorganic porous solids, and the recently-reported biomimetic porous surfaces that mimic the structure of cactus spines. Most of them, Yaghi argues, are not as productive as MOFs in taking up water from low humidity air. Nevertheless, further research may of course explore all possibilities to find the best solution, not only for harvesting water, but also for purifying it, guaranteeing the achievement of one of the most important UN goals—achieving access to adequate and equitable sanitation and hygiene for all.

Directed evolution of selective enzymes

Directed evolution of enzymes received the 2018 Nobel Prize in Chemistry. Enzymes produced through directed evolution are used to manufacture everything from biofuels to pharmaceuticals. According to the Nobel committee, chemists such as 2018 Laureate Frances H. Arnold "have taken control of evolution and used it for purposes that bring the greatest benefit to humankind." "Directed evolution requires the experimental testing of tens of thousands of variants, but [at the end] provides highly active enzymes," explains Sílvia Osuna, who investigates enzymes through advanced computational methods. She believes that the most active enzymes created through rational design "still perform quite poorly in comparison with the natural enzymes and enzymes artificially evolved in the lab." According to Osuna, the most interesting fact about directed evolution is how "mutations [that are] remote from the enzyme active site have a tremendous effect on the enzyme catalytic activity."

It is only through analyzing artificially evolved enzymes that we have come to learn this. Her field, studying enzymes through computation, could be the key to identifying similar trends, thus better understand directed evolution. "Computation is one of the many tools, together with protein engineering advances, gene synthesis, sequence analysis, and bioinformatics, that will help us chemists make more focused [enzyme] libraries," she concludes.

The limits of directed evolution are yet to be discovered. In her most recent paper, Arnold "hacked" plant enzyme cytochrome P450 using directed evolution. Now, they can easily catalyze the transformation carbon–hydrogen bonds into the more complicated asymmetric carbon–carbon bonds.

From plastics to monomers

"Circular economy is certainly the goal," says Tanja Junkers. Once again, chemists should be inspired by nature. There, "everything is reused, and we should do the same with our synthetic materials." This strategy will kill two birds with one stone, "it will solve the problem of recyclability in the long term, and the [need of] finding suitable sources for the main [polymer] building blocks."

Some polymers, like polylactic acid (PLA), can be easily recycled into their monomers just by using heat. Others, such as polyethylene-terephthalate (PET), can be similarly broken down into their most basic units. First, the polymer is treated with ethylene glycol, which breaks the long polymer chains down into oligomers. These smaller fragments melt at lower temperatures and therefore can be filtered to remove any impurities. Then, once the material has been purified, it's completely broken down into the monomers, which are then purified again by distillation.

Beyond classic chemistry, and much like Arnold's approach to enzymatic transformations noted earlier, some bacteria have evolved such that they can also break down PET into pieces. Sometimes plastic is the only source of carbon around and you need to adapt if you want to survive. At least one species of Nocardia possesses an esterase that can break the ester bonds in PET and, more recently, Japanese researchers discovered Ideonella sakaiensis, a bacterium that can disintegrate a PET plastic film in about six weeks thanks to two different enzymes. Yet, recycling is expensive, and "the world of plastics works on so small margins that every cent matter," says Junkers. Chemists are looking into cheaper options towards a circular economy. Moreover, the price of plastic will slowly rise as oil becomes less abundant. But, beyond that, we have to raise awareness that cleaner plastic may be more expensive, but worth it. "Society must be willing to pay a [higher] price for more sustainable options," concludes Junkers.

Reversible-deactivation of radical polymerization

"Reversible-deactivation of radical polymerizations (RDRP) was invented more than twenty years ago and revolutionized the world of polymers," explains Junkers. "These methods all rely on mechanisms that impose control over otherwise almost uncontrollable chain reactions, allowing us to design polymers with an accuracy that comes close to what nature is doing," she says. RDRP polymers have found uses in a myriad of sectors: construction, printing, energy, automotive, aerospace, and biomedical devices are just some examples. "Most of the time, we are using these polymers without realizing it," says Junkers. RDRP has become a very powerful and useful tool for industrial chemists.

But there is still plenty of room for further innovation, especially towards finding more environmentally-friendly polymerization solutions. There are now many methods to control RDRP processes using only light, even without the need of using metals [18]. In recent years, chemists have also developed RDRP methods that work in flow systems, which will allow them to move towards greener synthesis of polymers and plastics.

Finally, chemists have also mastered polymerization processes that work in aqueous media, avoiding the use of volatile or hazardous solvents. The most recent advances allow them to obtain ultra-high-molecular-weight polymers in water in just a few minutes, while keeping an exquisite control of the polymer branching. Some of these processes can work with a very low-energy light source, even just sunlight in some cases. Despite being a well-established technique, we can be certain that RDRP methods will continue to innovate, yielding an even broader commercial success.

3D-bioprinting

Bioprinting is one of today's most promising technologies. Using 3D printers and inks made out of living cells and also biomaterials and growth factors, chemists and biologists have managed to fabricate artificial tissues and organs almost indistinguishable from their natural versions. 3D-bioprinting could revolutionize both diagnostics and treatments, as artificial tissues and organs could be easily used for drug screening and toxicology research. This technology could even lead to the creation of tissues and organs for ideal transplants that would not require a donor. Currently, scientists can already 3D-print tubular tissues (heart, urethra, blood vessels), viscous organs (pancreas) and solid systems (bones). Recently, Cambridge researchers even managed to 3D-print a retina, carefully depositing layers of different types of living cells to generate a construct that architecturally resembles the native eye tissue.

Chemistry plays a central role in all the steps of this very complex process. First, organs and tissues need to be "scanned" in order to have a computational model. This is done using imaging techniques like computerized tomography (CT) scans and magnetic resonance imaging (MRI), both of which usually require chemical contrast agents such as gadolinium dyes. Then, bioprinting itself requires a myriad of chemicals to stabilize the bio-inks, trigger the assembly of the cells, or act as a scaffold for the printed tissue.

And finally, the 3D-bioprinted object needs to maintain its structure and form over time, a process for which both physical and chemical stimuli are required. Moreover, much like in any transplant or surgery, there is always the risk of the body rejecting the printed tissues. Understanding the chemistry of cell-cell recognition, mostly ruled by sugars that coat the membrane in the form of glycolipids and glycoproteins, is key to minimize rejection. Chemistry, in the center of all the crossing disciplines behind the highly-complex 3D-bioprinting, will be key in the further development of this fringe technique that, according to some experts, could even build new organs that are better than the existing biological ones

21. Conclusion

The consequences of chemistry are far-reaching. Chemistry has been largely responsible for shaping society as we know it; from developing stronger materials for large scale construction you use every day. Society has benefited hugely from advances in the field, with the few key discoveries outlined here just a small cross-section of the chemical innovations that have driven society's development. While discoveries in chemistry have made a huge impact, and continue to have enormous potential, we also need to ensure that we use them responsibly to ensure sustainability into the future. Chemistry could be an elementary and sanctioning science that investigates molecules—the building blocks of all matter—and however, they move to have an effect on the composition, structure and properties of drugs. The industrial applications of chemistry directly have an effect on our daily lives—what we tend to eat, what we tend to wear, our transport, the technology we tend to use, however, we tend to treat diseases and the way we tend to get electricity—to name simply a couple of. Research is consistently deepening our understanding of chemistry and resulting in new discoveries.

Today, research in chemistry is hugely diverse and involves areas as different as the monitoring and removal of pollutants from the atmosphere; the study of chromosomes, genes, and DNA replication; investigation of polysaccharides that decorate the surface of cells; elucidation of the role of small molecules in cell signaling; the production, conversion, and storage of energy; research on photosynthesis; the development of fertilizers that help produce rich harvests; and the continuing research on the creation of new materials for nanotechnology and for medical applications.

The many applications of chemistry in our lives have created a broad range of opportunities for employment. Chemistry is an integral part of the nation's economy, and the central discipline in several major industries. With B.Sc. degree in chemistry, students may find a research or technical position in a variety of industries such as oil, chemical, food processing, agriculture, photography, pharmaceuticals, biotechnology, mining, and others. In addition to the research, manufacturing, and diagnostic side of private employment, graduates with knowledge of chemistry work in sales and plant development, quality control, customer relations, and many other aspects of modern business. Students who combine a strong basic background in chemistry with further studies in business administration will find many opportunities in management, development, and administration available to them.

Combining the bachelor's degree in chemistry or chemical biology with a higher degree in another field can lead to many unique and rewarding careers. The B.A. in chemistry or B.S. in chemical biology is particularly useful for those who are interested in medicine and a professional career in medical research. A chemistry B.A. with a law degree can create a career in environmental or patent law. For students who wants to make research in chemistry a primary occupation, however, a higher degree in chemistry is essential. A Ph.D. in chemistry can lead to careers in academics, private industry, and government research laboratories.

The nation's concern about energy, the environment, and the detection of hazardous substances has added to the government's need for informed technical opinions on these subjects. The large national laboratories and many smaller ones provide constant opportunities for Ph.D. chemists to help shape the country's future in these crucial areas.